HEALTH CARE IN TRANSITION

MEDICAL CARE

PAST, PRESENT AND FUTURE PERSPECTIVES

HEALTH CARE IN TRANSITION

Additional books and e-books in this series can be found on Nova's website under the Series tab.

HEALTH CARE IN TRANSITION

MEDICAL CARE

PAST, PRESENT AND FUTURE PERSPECTIVES

BRIAN A. SOILEAU
EDITOR

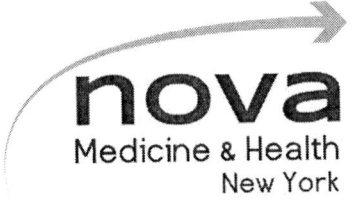

Copyright © 2020 by Nova Science Publishers, Inc.

All rights reserved. No part of this book may be reproduced, stored in a retrieval system or transmitted in any form or by any means: electronic, electrostatic, magnetic, tape, mechanical photocopying, recording or otherwise without the written permission of the Publisher.

We have partnered with Copyright Clearance Center to make it easy for you to obtain permissions to reuse content from this publication. Simply navigate to this publication's page on Nova's website and locate the "Get Permission" button below the title description. This button is linked directly to the title's permission page on copyright.com. Alternatively, you can visit copyright.com and search by title, ISBN, or ISSN.

For further questions about using the service on copyright.com, please contact:
Copyright Clearance Center
Phone: +1-(978) 750-8400   Fax: +1-(978) 750-4470   E-mail: info@copyright.com.

NOTICE TO THE READER

The Publisher has taken reasonable care in the preparation of this book, but makes no expressed or implied warranty of any kind and assumes no responsibility for any errors or omissions. No liability is assumed for incidental or consequential damages in connection with or arising out of information contained in this book. The Publisher shall not be liable for any special, consequential, or exemplary damages resulting, in whole or in part, from the readers' use of, or reliance upon, this material. Any parts of this book based on government reports are so indicated and copyright is claimed for those parts to the extent applicable to compilations of such works.

Independent verification should be sought for any data, advice or recommendations contained in this book. In addition, no responsibility is assumed by the Publisher for any injury and/or damage to persons or property arising from any methods, products, instructions, ideas or otherwise contained in this publication.

This publication is designed to provide accurate and authoritative information with regard to the subject matter covered herein. It is sold with the clear understanding that the Publisher is not engaged in rendering legal or any other professional services. If legal or any other expert assistance is required, the services of a competent person should be sought. FROM A DECLARATION OF PARTICIPANTS JOINTLY ADOPTED BY A COMMITTEE OF THE AMERICAN BAR ASSOCIATION AND A COMMITTEE OF PUBLISHERS.

Additional color graphics may be available in the e-book version of this book.

Library of Congress Cataloging-in-Publication Data

Names: Soileau, Brian A., editor.
Title: Medical care: past, present and future perspectives / [edited by] Brian A. Soileau.
Identifiers: LCCN 2020025138 (print) | LCCN 2020025139 (ebook) |
  ISBN 9781536180480 (paperback) | ISBN 9781536181043 (adobe pdf)
Subjects: LCSH: Medicine--Research. | Chronic diseases. | Fibromyalgia. | Rett syndrome.
Classification: LCC R850 .M34 2020 (print) | LCC R850 (ebook) | DDC 610.72--dc23
LC record available at https://lccn.loc.gov/2020025138
LC ebook record available at https://lccn.loc.gov/2020025139

Published by Nova Science Publishers, Inc. † New York

CONTENTS

Preface vii

Chapter 1 New Perspectives on the Pathophysiological Mechanisms of Fibromyalgia through Sensory Integration and Their Impact on the Quality of Daily Life 1
Patricija Goubar and Tomaž Velnar

Chapter 2 The Importance for Improvement of the Existing GMFM Score in Neurological Disorders 33
Alen Kapel, Tine Kovacic, Natasa Kos and Tomaz Velnar

Chapter 3 The Interdisciplinary Approach in the Rehabilitation of Patients with Rett Syndrome 51
Alen Kapel, Tine Kovacic, Tomaz Velnar and Natasa Kos

Chapter 4	The Role of Endplate in Degenerative Disc Disease Treatment: The Isolation of Human Chondrocytes from Vertebral Endplate *Lidija Gradisnik, Uros Maver, Gorazd Bunc, Matjaz Vorsic, Janez Ravnik, Tomaz Smigoc, Roman Bosnjak and Tomaz Velnar*	**71**
Chapter 5	The Degenerative Disease of Intervertebral Disc and Surgical Results after Microsurgical Discectomy *Lidija Gradisnik, Tomaz Velnar and Gorazd Bunc*	**95**
Index		**113**

Preface

*Medical Care: Past, Present and Future Perspective*s first presents important research regarding the fibromyalgia may be a possible pathophysiological mechanisms of fibromyalgia. Current research suggests that the basis for modified physiology of the central nervous system, with the nature of changes in the brain directing the thinking that fibromyalgia could be a primary brain disease.

Next, in order to examine the effects of complex interdisciplinary neurophysiotherapy, five girls with Rett syndrome were included in an experimental study to assess gross motor function before and after habilitation.

Rett syndrome is a rare genetic neurological syndrome, affecting almost only females and leading to severe impairments in all areas of the affected persons' life, including speech, mobility, posture, digestive and pulmonary function.

Subsequently, in order to study the degenerative processes of endplate chondrocytes in vitro, the authors present a relatively quick and easy protocol for the isolation of human chondrocytes from vertebral endplates.

In closing, the mechanisms of the intervertebral disc degeneration and associated factors are presented, as well as short-term surgical results with microdiscectomy treatment.

Chapter 1 - Fibromyalgia (FM) is a syndrome of chronic and widespread musculoskeletal pain with a wide range of symptoms, including chronic fatigue, sleep disturbances, difficulties with memory, poor concentration, and mood swings. The pathophysiological mechanism of FM has been linked to central and peripheral nervous system dysfunction. However, the exact pathophysiological mechanism is still unknown, especially the role of multisensory hypersensitivity in affected individuals and its effects on daily life. The purpose of the authors' study was to determine whether individuals with FM had increased levels of sensory defensiveness and consequently decreased quality of daily life and to explore their correlations. Female patients with FM were compared with healthy pain-free individuals (controls). An independent, randomly selected sample of 71 subjects was used. 34 patients with at least one year diagnosed with FM based on the American College of Rheumatology (ACR) diagnostic criteria were classified into the fibromyalgia (FM group) and 37 patients without FM were placed in the control group. Research included a quantitative, cross-sectional study using two questionnaires: a self-report measure of sensory sensitivity to stimuli present in daily life (Adult/Adolescent Sensory Profile) and an evaluation of the health-related quality of daily life (The Short form – 36 Health Survey, version 2). Data was used to determine differences between groups using the nonparametric Mann–Whitney test for two samples and when using the ordinal dependent variable Chi-square test. Statistically significant differences were confirmed for p values less than 0.05. It was found that female patients with FM reported significantly more symptoms related to sensory deficiency the presence and degree of sensory sensitivity in the FM group was significantly higher than in the control group, and there was a statistically significant difference between the groups ($p < 0.0001$). Additionally, this group experienced more stress in daily life, as its constituents have a statistically significant lower quality of life in the assessment of physical health ($p < 0.0001$), mental health ($p < 0.0001$), and social functioning ($p = 0.022$) than the healthy people in the control group. Based on the authors' findings, this review of the paper presents important points about the possible pathophysiological mechanism of fibromyalgia.

Current research suggests that the basis for FM may be a modified physiology of the central nervous system, with the nature of changes in the brain directing the thinking that fibromyalgia could be a primary brain disease.

Chapter 2 - Despite many various scores and ways of assessment that have been developed so far for the evaluation of motor functions in persons with special needs, there is still no perfect score existing. Gross Motor Function Measure is a useful scale for evaluating the gross motor function of persons with special needs. There are two versions of the GMFM in use, the 66 and 88. They differ in the types of disorders being used for. In this study, the authors propose an improved version of the GMFM score, including movement quality, quality of locomotor execution and postural characteristics. An improved version of the GMFM was tested by neurophysiotherapists in five girls with Rett syndrome. The improved version was also examined by 49 neurophysotherapist and 19 doctors. Although the GMFM-88 provides key factors in subject's gross motor function status, it is not able to provide or evaluate the quality of motor ability concerning movement, execution and transition quality, multidimensional movement and postural characteristics in sitting and standing position. The results confirmed that the modified GMFM-88, including all these parameters, was a valid and reliable instrument for evaluating gross motor function for a specific group of neurological disorders. These new elements are thus essential factors added in the modified GMFM and form a part of a more thorough multidisciplinary interventional approach in the treatment of Rett syndrome patients.

Chapter 3 - Rett syndrome is a rare genetic neurological syndrome, affecting almost only females and leading to severe impairments in all areas of the affected persons' life, including speech, mobility, posture, digestive and pulmonary function. Most distinct symptoms include stereotypical hand movements, ataxia and atrophy of lower limbs and signs of autism. The neurological disorders in patients with Rett syndrome embrace various types of impairments or abnormalities, underlined by biochemical and structural abnormalities of brain, spinal cord and peripheral nerves. Clinically, these conditions may involve several disorders, including paralysis, spasticity, seizures, orthopaedic deformities, pain syndromes, disturbances of coordination, mobility and others. An interdisciplinary approach to neurological disorders demonstrated in Rett syndrome is therefore of utmost importance. The aim is to revert progressive deterioration with a wide spectrum and a combination of neurorehabilitational interventions. In order to examine the effects of complex interdisciplinary neurophysiotherapy, five girls with Rett syndrome were included in the authors' experimental study. The GMFM-88 scale was used to determine the gross motor function prior and after habilitation. It was found that the interdisciplinary approach with combined neurophysiotherapy and continuous habilitation was very efficient in the gross motor function improvement in these patients, which has confirmed the importance of an interdisciplinary approach in the habilitation of the disease symptoms.

Chapter 4 - *Introduction.* As a replacement option for laboratory animals, the *in vitro* organ culture systems are becoming increasingly essential. To study the possible mechanisms of intervertebral disc (IVD) degeneration, live disc cells are highly appealing. Especially the endplate plays an essential role in the degenerative disc disease. Although most intervertebral disc cells have been isolated from animal tissue, the experimental result cannot be conveyed from animals directly to humans. In order to study the degenerative processes of the endplate chondrocytes in vitro, the authors have established a relatively quick and easy protocol for isolation of human chondrocytes from the vertebral endplates.

Materials and Methods. The fragments of human lumbar endplate were obtained following lumbar fusion. The cartilaginous endplate fragments were collected, cut, grinded and partially digested with collagenase I. Sequential centrifugation and separation followed after enzymatic digestion, then the sediment was harvested and cells were seeded in suspension, supplemented with special media containing high nutrient level. Morphology was determined with phalloidin staining and the characterization for collagen I, collagen II and aggrecan with immunostaining.

Results. In appropriate laboratory conditions, the isolated cells retained viability and proliferated quickly. The confluent culture was obtained after 14 days. Six to 8 hours after seeding, attachments were observed and after 12 hours, proliferation of the isolated cells followed. The cartilaginous endplate chondrocytes were stable with the viability up to 95%.

Conclusion. Human chondrocyte cell culture allows the *in vitro* study of endplate cells. The reported cell isolation process is simple, economical and quick, allowing establishing a viable long-term cell culture. The availability of chondrocyte cell model will permit the study of cell properties, biochemical aspects, the potential of therapeutic candidates for the treatment of disc degeneration as well as toxicology studies in a well-controlled environment.

Chapter 5 - The degenerative disease of the intervertebral disc and back pain are chronic conditions that are frequently encountered in clinical practice, especially in young and active population. They are caused by numerous factors and represent an important cause of both morbidity and mortality. Patient comorbidities and numerous associated risk factors may contribute to the onset of the degenerative process. Several factors play a role in the degenerative disc disease, which most commonly affects the nucleus pulposus and eventually influences the biomechanics of the spine. The consequences of the degenerative disc disease are among the main initiative factors for chronic instability of the diseased spinal segments and result in functional disability in both sexes, significantly affecting the quality of living. The mechanisms of the intervertebral disc degeneration and associated factors are presented, as well as the authors' short-term surgical results with microdiscectomy treatment.

In: Medical Care
Editor: Brian A. Soileau

ISBN: 978-1-53618-048-0
© 2020 Nova Science Publishers, Inc.

Chapter 1

New Perspectives on the Pathophysiological Mechanisms of Fibromyalgia through Sensory Integration and Their Impact on the Quality of Daily Life

Patricija Goubar[1], and Tomaž Velnar[2],†*
[1]Department of Health Sciences,
Alma Mater Europaea – ECM, Maribor, Slovenia
[2]Department of Neurosurgery, University Medical Centre Ljubljana,
Ljubljana, Slovenia

Abstract

Fibromyalgia (FM) is a syndrome of chronic and widespread musculoskeletal pain with a wide range of symptoms, including chronic fatigue, sleep disturbances, difficulties with memory, poor concentration,

---

* Corresponding Author's Email: patricija.goubar@almamater.si.
† Corresponding Author's Email: tvelnar@hotmail.com.

and mood swings. The pathophysiological mechanism of FM has been linked to central and peripheral nervous system dysfunction. However, the exact pathophysiological mechanism is still unknown, especially the role of multisensory hypersensitivity in affected individuals and its effects on daily life. The purpose of our study was to determine whether individuals with FM had increased levels of sensory defensiveness and consequently decreased quality of daily life and to explore their correlations. Female patients with FM were compared with healthy pain-free individuals (controls). An independent, randomly selected sample of 71 subjects was used. 34 patients with at least one year diagnosed with FM based on the American College of Rheumatology (ACR) diagnostic criteria were classified into the fibromyalgia (FM group) and 37 patients without FM were placed in the control group. Research included a quantitative, cross-sectional study using two questionnaires: a self-report measure of sensory sensitivity to stimuli present in daily life (Adult/Adolescent Sensory Profile) and an evaluation of the health-related quality of daily life (The Short form – 36 Health Survey, version 2). Data was used to determine differences between groups using the nonparametric Mann–Whitney test for two samples and when using the ordinal dependent variable Chi-square test. Statistically significant differences were confirmed for p values less than 0.05. It was found that female patients with FM reported significantly more symptoms related to sensory deficiency the presence and degree of sensory sensitivity in the FM group was significantly higher than in the control group, and there was a statistically significant difference between the groups ($p < 0.0001$). Additionally, this group experienced more stress in daily life, as its constituents have a statistically significant lower quality of life in the assessment of physical health ($p < 0.0001$), mental health ($p < 0.0001$), and social functioning ($p = 0.022$) than the healthy people in the control group. Based on our findings, this review of the paper presents important points about the possible pathophysiological mechanism of fibromyalgia. Current research suggests that the basis for FM may be a modified physiology of the central nervous system, with the nature of changes in the brain directing the thinking that fibromyalgia could be a primary brain disease.

Keywords: fibromyalgia, sensory integration, central modulation, quality of life, sensory hypersensitivity

INTRODUCTION

Fibromyalgia syndrome (FMS) is a common chronic pain syndrome characterized by unexplained idiopathic, widespread pain (Mease 2005, 6). The pathophysiological mechanism of FMS is associated with central and peripheral nervous system dysfunction (Brietzke et al. 2019, 1-2). It affects about 2% of the adult population in the United States and other regions of the world where FMS is being studied. More than 90% of patients are women (Wilbarger and Cook 2011, 653). Prevalence in certain regions has not been established and may be influenced by differences in cultural norms regarding the definition of chronic pain conditions (Mease 2005, 6). A fundamental feature of FMS is chronic and widespread musculoskeletal pain, which lasts for at least three months; other symptoms include sleep disorders, chronic fatigue, irritable bowel and bladder, chronic headache, visual disturbances, memory disorders, concentration disorders, and mood disorders (Brietzke et al. 2019, 7; Mease 2005, 6; Wilbarger and Cook 2011; 653). For many years, fibromyalgia has not been properly defined and properly addressed, even though it is an old disease that was historically considered an emotional and psychosomatic disorder or a particular form of depression (Wolfe et al. 2010, 600-1). It was initially classified as fibrositis syndrome (Smythe and Moldofsky 1977, 928). Only after the publication of the first study by Smythe and Moldofsky (1977) and the first call for diagnostic criteria did fibromyalgia research gain high levels of interest, provoking more than sixty studies that increased clinical acceptance and validation of the syndrome (Bennett 1981, 405; Smythe and Moldofsky 1977, 928; Yunus et al. 1981, 151; Yunus et al. 1989, 69; Wolfe 1986, 99). In 1987, the American Medical Association (AMA) named FMS an independent form of the disease, notwithstanding the fact that international diagnostic criteria were only adopted in 1990 at the American College of Rheumatology (ACR) (Wolfe et al. 1990, 160). The World Health Organization (WHO) confirmed FMS as an independent form of the disease in 1993 (Chaitow 2003, 1). The clinical diagnostic criteria were initially based on defining the number of pressure-positive pain points on the muscles and musculoskeletal areas, where even a light touch can provoke a strong pain response. Eleven out of eighteen such points in the presence of pain for at least three months and with sleep disturbances are thought to be sensitive to clinical diagnosis (Wolfe et al. 1990, 171; Buskila et al. 1997, 238-40). A decade later, the criteria for clinical diagnosis in 1990 were no longer optimal and were completely revised at ACR in 2010. A number of rheumatologists have adopted the new diagnostic criteria. as valid criteria for determining the diagnosis of FMS (Yunus and Aldag 2012, 71-5). The new criteria are considered by the experts to be significantly more useful as they enable easier and more objective diagnoses by omitting the identification of pain points, which were often based on subjective assessment. Criteria for assessing the prevalence of pain, the severity of symptoms, and many other disease signs were added to the new criteria. An advantage is the ability to monitor the course of the disease, especially its variability in symptoms. Experts note that, according to new criteria, the reliability of diagnosis is extremely high, accounting for as much as 88.1% (Wolfe et al. 2010, 600-9). Diagnostic criteria help to understand this patient population and, at the same time, the multidimensional nature of this syndrome (Clauw and Crofford 2003, 685-700). Although the etiology of FMS is not fully understood, it is believed that the syndrome results from the influence of various factors, such as genetic relatedness, stress, chronic diseases, and various pain conditions, which in some but not all patients are associated with various disorders of neurotransmitters function and neuroendocrine disorders (Montoya et al. 2006, 1995-8). The unifying assumption is that FMS stems from central nervous system sensitivity. Namely, recent research has highlighted a number of potential underlying neurophysiological disorders, based primarily on a lower tolerance threshold for pain perception or over-sensitivity in different sensory systems in patients with FMS as compared to patients who do not develop the syndrome (Cook et al. 2004, 364-5; Kosek et al. 1996, 375-81). Increased sensitivity to somatosensory stimuli is associated with differences in brain activity in patients with FMS compared to a healthy population as measured by magnetic resonance imaging (MR) and electroencephalographic muscle activity (EEG) (Gracely et al. 2002,

1333). Hypersensitivity findings to sensory stimuli in both psychophysiological as well as neurological studies have contributed to a number of FMS-related theories, including poor central modulation of nociception, generalized higher excitability to sensory stimuli, and general central nervous system sensitivity. Such findings and arguments have great weight in defining the daily quality of life of patients with FMS, who often report the presence of sensitivity, even pain, and unusual sensations to somatic and non-somatic stimuli such as pressure, electrical and thermal stimuli, or light touch, certain sounds, and odours in everyday life (Ubago Linares et al. 2008, 613-17; Wilbarger and Cook 2011, 653). The presence of such sensitivities may, in addition to the underlying pain symptomatology, further contribute to difficulties in the daily functioning of the patient and to the creation of an additional source of stress, anxiety, and fatigue (Wilbarger and Cook 2011, 653-4).

The first definition of sensory integration was first set in 1979 by Anna Jean Ayres, PhD in Psychology, a neuroscientist and occupational therapist, who began working on the process of sensory integration in 1960 (Ayres 1987, 93; Smith Roley et al. 2007, 2-3). Sensory integration theory has been defined by Anna Jean Ayres as an unconscious neurological process that takes place in our brains. It is responsible for receiving and organizing sensory information from the body and the environment, further for filtering and classifying that information into important and irrelevant, thus enabling the appropriate response of the individual's body and its adaptation and functioning within its environment (Schaaf and Mailloux 2015, 5). The sensory system is a part of the larger neurological system, which is responsible for the proper processing of sensory information. Its composition encompasses many sensory neurons, neural pathways, and individual brain areas that are involved in sensory perception (Bundy et al. 2002, 36-43). Good central sensory integration is primarily the responsibility of the central nervous system. The individual centres in the central nervous system must interact, cooperate and act in concert. The stimuli are received by the receptors in the senses. There they are converted into electrical impulses that travel along the neuro-pathways to the brain. The central nervous system receives, adapts, connects, and organizes information (Miller et al. 2007, 136-8; Bundy et al. 2002, 36-43). Sensory integration encompasses the interaction of seven systems, namely: visual, auditory, gustatory and olfactory, tactile, vestibular and proprioception (Smith Roley et al. 2007, 3). The stimuli that come into our brains through these sensory systems are some kind of transducers that transmit information from the body or from the environment to the brain, whereupon they are processed for the appropriate adaptive response or for our own perception of the environment around us; they further store the experience for later use when needed. This part of the system is therefore referred to as the associative or integrative nervous system (Schwartz and Krantz 2019, 17-9; Bundy et al. 2002, 10-2). Integration means the effective composition and organization of sensory information as a whole, in the central nervous system, into which at every moment arrive a great deal of new impulses, which are fundamental for gaining new experiences for optimal daily functioning (Ayres 2005, 6-8). Sensory integration dysfunction indicates abnormalities in various segments of the neurological system, which has a direct impact on the effective organization and successful integration of various sensory inflows (Miller et al. 2007, 135-7). In the categorization of sensory processing disorders, we refer to disorders in three areas, namely: sensory modulation disorder (regulation), sensory discrimination disorder (recognition), and sensory motor disorder (movement and skill). To the extent that there is a disturbance in the registration or modulation of sensory stimuli, this is reflected in various forms of sensitivity and responsiveness (Ayres 1966, 741-4; Miller et al. 2007, 136-7). Sensory modulation is divided into three subgroups. The first involves sensory hypersensitivity or hypersensitivity in the form of either an excessively intense or long response to a particular stimulus, or a response to a very low intensity stimulus. The second group includes insufficient sensory sensitivity, indicating inadequate response to a stimulus, or a response only to an extremely strong stimulus. The third group includes sensory search for individual inflows or the search for an increasing number of powerful stimuli (Ayres 1966, 741-4; Bundy et al. 2002, 102-14). A key finding of many authors and researchers is the high proportion of the presence of sensory integration disorder in persons with

FMS (Dixon et al. 2016, 537-8; Blumentstiel et al. 2011, 682-90; Geisser et al. 2008, 235-42; Smith et al. 2008, 420-8). Of particular importance to the FMS is the disturbance in the sensory modulation, which includes the difficulty in organizing a response related to sensory inflow or information in regarding to the reduced ability to regulate and thus inappropriate response to the sensory environment. It is manifested as excessive sensitivity to stimuli or hypersensitivity and often as withdrawal from stimuli (Brietzke et al. 2019, 6). Sensory modulation disorder in FMS is expressed through a reduced threshold of perception of discomfort or pain due to somatic stimuli such as pressure, electrical stimuli, and thermal stimuli (Geisser et al. 2008, 417-8; Gracely et al. 2002, 1333-43; Kosek et al. 1996, 375-6). These patients typically report discomfort or pain at a lower stimulus intensity level than do healthy subjects (Kosek et al. 1996, 375-83). The proportion of patients with FMS also reported discomfort with exposure to non-somatic stimuli such as sound (Geisser et al. 2002, 1333; Carrillo-de-la Pena et al. 2006, 480). Since optimal sensory modulation means the ability to regulate sensory stimuli to respond appropriately to the sensory environment, and thus also means the individual's well-being, in addition to the already present multidimensional FMS symptom, it certainly has an additional impact on FMS patients through their daily functioning in work, social, or home environments (Schoen et al. 2014, 522; Salaffi et al. 2009; 67-74). Given the unknown etiology and broad dimension of FMS, a variety of medical procedures and approaches are used for treatment, including medication treatment, which often includes primarily antidepressants, opioids, non-steroidal anti-inflammatory drugs, sedatives or antidepressants, muscle relaxants, and antiepileptics. Non-pharmaceutical treatments, including aerobic exercise, physical therapy, massage, acupuncture, and cognitive behavioural therapy, may also be helpful (Goldenberg et al. 2004, 2389-92). Some of these approaches have been shown to have unambiguous benefits in the improvement of well-being and pain regulation, as well as of other symptoms in persons with FMS. However, interest in finding optimal treatment approaches, without side effects, is growing, as newer and more effective therapies are developed based on their ability to accurately measure the effect (Wilbarger and Cook 2011, 654). The complexity of FMS suggests that multimodal individual assessment and treatment programs are required to achieve optimal treatment results in patients with this syndrome (Goldenberg et al. 2004, 2393). In addition to the already established medication and physical therapy in the treatment of FMS, on the basis of numerous contemporary findings, research on FMS also raises proposals for the integration of Sensory Integration therapies, with the aim of influencing the ability to receive and respond to sensory stimuli, while improving the quality of daily functioning and the lives of subjects with FMS (Schoen et al. 2014, 522-30; Dixon et al. 2016, 537-50; Bernard et al. 2000, 42-9).

Considering all the starting points, the purpose of our study was to define the relationship and correlation between sensory modulation and quality of daily life in adults with FMS as compared with subjects without FMS. We predicted that subjects with FMS had a statistically significant higher presence and level of sensory hypersensitivity compared to subjects without FMS. For this reason, we further predicted that persons with FMS had a statistically significantly lower health-related daily quality of life compared to subjects without FMS.

METHODS

Design

The study was based on a quantitative research method conducted in the form of a randomized, comparative, cross-sectional study. It was performed at the Medical Centre for Sensory Integration in Slovenia, in cooperation with the Fibromyalgia Society of Slovenia and the International University of Alma Mater Europaea, European Centre Maribor. Before participating in the study, the participants signed an informed consent, the data are protected in accordance with the Personal Data Protection Act of the Republic of Slovenia and the General Data Protection Regulation (GDPR).

Participants

The study involved an independent, randomly selected research sample of 71 individuals, consisting of 27 men and 44 women, which were divided into two groups. 34 subjects with at least one-year FMS diagnose were classified in the fibromyalgia (FM) group and 37 subjects without FMS were classified in the control group. The FM group consisted of 12 men and 22 women diagnosed with FMS by doctors, based on the diagnostic criteria of the American College of Rheumatology (ACR). The subjects were selected at the Medical Centre for Sensory Integration of Slovenia and the Fibromyalgia Society of Slovenia. Their age ranged from 27 to 63 years, with an average age of 41.4 years. The control group included 15 men and 22 women. Their age range was 26 to 63 years, with an average age of 42.6 years. The overall mean age of all participants was 43 years (SD = 9.62). We excluded from testing all those with presenting conditions that coincide with similar symptoms to disorders of sensory modulation, or could have an impact on the final outcome of the quality of day-to-day assessment.

Instruments

The classification of the presence or absence of sensory modulation disorders was based on an assessment performed via a standardized Adolescent/Adult Sensory Profile Questionnaire. Furthermore, participants completed a standardized questionnaire to assess the health-related quality of daily life (The Short form – 36 Health Survey, version 2). Both questionnaires were completed after the informed consent was signed at the Sensory Integration Medical Centre.

The Adolescent/Adult Sensory Profile (AASP) standardized questionnaire is a self-assessment instrument for assessing the sensory profile of adolescents and adults 11 to 65+ years of age. It is a standardized method of self-assessment and the impact of sensory processing on daily functioning and response. It was developed from the basic Sensory Profile

Assessment Instrument (Dunn 1999), which identifies atypical processing of sensory inflow in children 3 to 10 years of age. AASP is easy to use because of its clear composition, with a lead time of 10 to 15 minutes. It consists of four quadrants, each including 15 questions, covering the following categories of sensory processing: Taste/Smell, Movement (vestibular and proprioceptive), Visual, Tactile and Auditory. In total, it consists of 60 statements describing responses to exposure to daily sensory experiences. The respondent can choose from answers on a 5-point rating scale (1-Almost Never, 2-Seldom, 3-Occasionally, 3-Frequently, 5-Almost Always). In the analysis, the sum of the individual statements pertaining to the different categories of sensory processing is calculated and the total sum of the points of all quadrants is calculated. Total sum is the most sensitive indicator of sensory dysfunction. The sums of the quadrants of each area fall into three categories: Low registration, Sensation Seeking, Sensory Sensitivity, and Sensation Avoiding (Dunn 1999; Dunn and Brown 2002; McIntosh et al. 1999, 608-15; Pearson Education 2008). In our study, based on a theoretical background, the FM group used data to characterize sensory modulation disorders in the direction of sensory sensitization and avoidance of stimuli, in a further analysis.

The Short form – 36 Health Survey, version 2 – The SF-36v2® (SF-36) is the most commonly used questionnaire to measure the quality of life of people with various disorders or illnesses. It is a multidimensional questionnaire that assesses health-related quality of life through individual scales. The SF-36 questionnaire indicates a short form derived from a four-year Medical Outcome Study (MOS), which examined the impact of disease characteristics, the health system, and patients themselves on the outcome of treatment. 36 questions of 149 were ultimately selected to be the best indicator of health-related quality of life. In terms of content, the questionnaire covers eight areas of health, which combine into two supercategories: the physical and the mental. The body component consists of the following scales: Body performance, Body performance limitations, Body pain, and General health. The mental component consists of the following scales: Mental health, Emotional problems, Social functioning, and Vitality. The questionnaire is standardized and validated in many countries, translated into 140 languages, using more than 17,000 clinical studies by the year of 2011. The authors of the SF-36 questionnaire provide high reliability of the individual scales. When collecting norms on the general American population in 2009 (N = 4024), the coefficients of reliability (alpha) ranged from 0.82 to 0.96. The results of the questionnaire are analysed using standard points (T), where higher scores mean better quality of life (Maruish 2011). For the purposes of the study, we used the results of three indicators of health-related quality of life in the analysis of questionnaire SF-36: physical health, mental health and social functioning.

Statistical Analysis

IBM SPSS Statistics 23 was used to process the data. For the basic data review, descriptive statistics were performed, looking at the mean, standard deviation of the median, and the minimum and maximum values of the variables. Some demographics were shown using frequencies and percentages. Before testing the hypotheses, we used the Shapiro–Wilk test to verify that our dependent numerical variables are normally distributed in all groups. Because we found that the distribution of dependent variables deviates from normal in at least one group, we used a nonparametric Mann–Whitney U test for two samples to determine differences between groups. When using the ordinal dependent variable, we calculated the Chi-square test, and we were also interested in the difference between the two groups. The research hypotheses were confirmed in cases where the statistical significance of each test was less than 0.05.

RESULTS

71 people were included in the survey, 47.9% of them with FMS, and 52.1% of the sample were persons without FMS. The average age of the

respondents is 43 years (SD = 9.62). The youngest respondent is 26 years and the oldest is 63 years old.

The following variables were used to test the first hypothesis: two were summarized from the AASP questionnaire Sensory Sensitivity and Avoidance of stimuli, and both groups of respondents (test and control group). Prior to testing, we verified using the Shapiro–Wilk test if the data (sensory sensitivity level and stimulus avoidance rate) were distributed normally according to the patient group. Based on the value of the statistical significance of the Shapiro–Wilk test, we found that the distribution of sensory sensitivity and stimulus avoidance rates across the group deviates from normal in both groups, since the statistical significance in both groups is less than 0.05 for both variables. We used the non-parametric Mann–Whitney test to determine differences between groups and, using descriptive statistics, found that sensory sensitivity was, on average, higher in subjects with FMS (M = 56.88; SD = 6.55) compared with subjects without FMS (M = 33.12; SD = 5.86). Considering the value of the statistical significance of the Mann–Whitney test, we find that there is a statistically significant difference between subjects without FMS and those with FMS in the level of sensory sensitivity (p <0.0001). Based on average values, we found that subjects with fibromyalgia had a higher degree of sensory sensitivity compared to subjects without FMS. Also, based on the average rank, we find that persons in the test group have a higher level of sensory sensitivity, since the average rank in this group of respondents is higher (Mean rank = 54.41). A statistically significant difference also existed between the groups in stimulus avoidance (p <0.0001). Based on the average values in the descriptive statistics and the average rank, it is evident that persons with fibromyalgia have a higher rate of avoidance of stimuli (Mean rank = 53.01) than those without FMS (Mean rank = 20.36).

Going forward we were interested in the question in which sensory systems in persons with FMS are the modulation disorders more pronounced. Upon a closer examination of the individual categories of

Table 1. Descriptive statistics and Mann–Whitney test to identify differences between test and control groups in sensory sensitivity and stimulus avoidance

Group		Descriptive statistics						Mann–Whitney test		
		N	Median	Mean	Std. Deviation	Minimum	Maximum	Mann–Whitney U	Mean Rank	p
3. Sensory sensitivity	Subjects with fibromyalgia	34	54.5	56.88	6.55	47	74	3.00	54.41	0.000
	Subjects without FMS	37	32.0	33.22	5.86	19	47		19.08	
4. Avoiding stimuli	Subjects with fibromyalgia	34	49.0	50.85	6.24	41	70	50.50	53.01	0.000
	Subjects without FMS	37	29.0	31.49	6.58	22	52		20.36	

sensory processing, through the analysis of data from the AASP questionnaire, we found in the test group that the highest deviations in the direction of sensitivity were mainly on the vestibular system (72.5%), which together with the proprioceptive system indicates the "Movement" category, followed by the visual system of the *Visual category* (68%). Meanwhile, the highest level of stimulus avoidance was found in the "Tactile" category, which indicates hypersensitivity and thus withdrawal of touch-related stimuli (69.3%), followed by the vestibular system of Movement category (65.1%). The fewest problems with hypersensitivity and stimulus avoidance in the test group in our sample are identified in the "Taste/Smell" category.

In the second part of the analysis, we examined the presence of sensory sensitivity and the avoidance of stimuli according to the group of subjects with FMS and the group of persons without FMS. The analysis was made using the chi-square test. The results of the contingency table show that the frequency of sensory sensitivity is significantly higher in most people with FMS compared to the control group (94.1%). Among the subjects in the control group, the majority (89.2%) have sensory sensitivity categorized as Similar to other people, while the categorization of most subjects in the FM group (94.1%) is "much more than other people", which is the most difficult classification of sensitization. Considering the value of statistical significance, we found that the difference in the presence of sensory sensitivity was statistically significant with respect to the test group of subjects with FMS and the control group ($p < 0.0001$). From the results in the second contingency table, we further found the presence of stimulus avoidance in most people with fibromyalgia as compared to other people in the control group (52.9%). Among 44.1% of those with FMS the aforementioned rate of stimulus avoidance was categorized as the most difficult classification of sensitization, namely, Much more than other people and among 52.9% More than other people. The control group showed that most people had no problems with hypersensitivity, as the survey results in most of them fall into the category Similar to other people (75.7%). We found a statistically significant difference in the presence of stimuli avoidance ($p < 0.0001$), depending on the test group of subjects with fibromyalgia and control subjects. Thus, based on the analysis, the first hypothesis, which states that subjects with FMS have a statistically higher presence and level of sensory sensitization as compared to subjects without FMS, was confirmed.

Table 2. Contingency tables for determining differences in the presence of sensory sensitivity and stimulus avoidance by test and control groups

		Sensory sensitivity			Avoiding stimuli		
		Group		Total	Group		Total
		Subjects with fibromyalgia	Subjects without FMS		Subjects with fibromyalgia	Subjects without FMS	
Less than other people	Count	0	1	1	0	7	7
	%	0.0%	2.7%	1.4%	0.0%	18.9%	9.9%
Similar than other people	Count	0	33	33	1	28	29
	%	0.0%	89.2%	46.5%	2.9%	75.7%	40.8%
More than other people	Count	2	3	5	18	1	19
	%	5.9%	8.1%	7.0%	52.9%	2.7%	26.8%
Much more than other people	Count	32	0	32	15	1	16
	%	94.1%	0.0%	45.1%	44.1%	2.7%	22.5%
Total	Count	34	37	71	34	37	71
	%	100.0%	100.0%	100.0%	100.0%	100.0%	100.0%

Table 3. Chi-square test results

	Sensory sensitivity			Avoiding stimuli		
	Value	df	p	Value	df	p
Pearson Chi-Square	66.191[a]	3	0.000	59.578[b]	3	0.000
N	71			71		

[a] 4 cells (50.0%) have expected count less than 5. The minimum expected count is 0.48.
[b] 2 cells (25.0%) have expected count less than 5. The minimum expected count is 3.35.

Below, we compared the quality of life between the two groups. For verification, we again used the data of only three SF-36 indicators to determine health-related quality of life. We used the variables Physical health, Mental health, and Social functioning, along with both groups, test and control. Before testing the hypothesis, we used the Shapiro–Wilk test again to test whether the data (physical health, mental health, social functioning) were distributed normally according to the patient group (test and control group). Depending on the value of the statistical feature of the Shapiro–Wilk test, it can be seen that the distribution of the assessment of physical health, mental health and social functioning deviates from the normal in at least one group (FM group, control group), since the value of the statistical characteristic is at least in one group for each dependent variable less than 0.05. A non-parametric Mann–Whitney test was used to determine the differences between the groups in assessing physical, mental health, and social functioning. Using descriptive statistics, we found that, on average, physical health scores were better for people without FMS (M = 74.53; SD = 15.60) than for people with FMS (M = 35.74; SD = 15.08). Mental health was also found to be, on average, better for the control group respondents (M = 71.46; SD = 13.37) than for the FM group (M = 27.06; SD = 12.26). And last but not least, social functioning is, on average, slightly better for the respondents in the control group (M = 52.36; SD = 7.70) than for the subjects with FMS in the FM group (M = 48.16; SD = 6.97). Based on the value of the Mann–Whitney statistical significance test, we found that there was a statistically significant difference between subjects without FMS in the control group and those with FMS in the FM group in the assessment of physical health ($p < 0.0001$), mental health ($p < 0.0001$), and social functioning ($p = 0.022$). Based on the descriptive statistics and the higher average rank in the control group, we found that subjects without FMS have statistically significant better physical health, mental health, and better social functioning than subjects with FMS. Therefore, they could be said to have a better health-related quality of daily life. The second hypothesis, which states that subjects with FMS have a statistically significantly lower quality of daily living compared to subjects without FMS, is confirmed on the basis of the analysis.

Table 4. Descriptive statistics and Mann–Whitney test to determine quality of life differences between test and control group

Group		Descriptive statistics						Mann–Whitney test		
		N	Median	Mean	Std. Deviation	Minimum	Maximum	Mann-Whitney U	Mean Rank	p
Physical health	Subjects with fibromyalgia	34	35.0	35.74	15.08	5.0	70.0	61.5	19.31	0.000
	Subjects without FMS	37	80.0	74.32	15.60	35.0	95.0		51.34	
	Total	71	55.0	55.85	24.68	5.0	95.0			
Mental heath	Subjects with fibromyalgia	34	26.0	27.06	12.26	0.0	48.0	12.5	17.87	0.000
	Subjects without FMS	37	72.0	71.46	13.37	32.0	96.0		52.66	
	Total	71	52.0	5020	25.73	0.0	96.0			
Social functioning	Subjects with fibromyalgia	34	50.0	48.16	6.97	37.5	62.5	464.5	31.16	0.022
	Subjects without FMS	37	50.0	52.36	7.70	37.5	75.0		40.45	
	Total	71	50.0	50.35	7.61	37.5	75.0			

Conclusion

Sensory integration dysfunction (SID) is common in people with FMS, which, according to many authors, may have an additional impact on their quality of life (Kosek et al. 1996, 379-81; Mendoza-Battle 2014, 20-9; Miller et al. 2017; Salaffi et al. 2009, 67-73; Wilbarger and Cook 2011, 653-5; Zimmer and Desch 2012, 1186-9). We also predicted in our study that people with FMS had a significantly poorer ability to receive and respond to stimuli from the sensory environment, and the associated statistically significant lower quality of daily life compared to people without FMS. We have confirmed the predictions, as we found that SID in people with fibromyalgia defines abnormalities primarily in sensory modulation problems, which are manifested by marked over-sensitivity and/or withdrawal to a single stimulus compared with people without FMS. In addition to the multidimensional symptoms of fibromyalgia, both additionally impact the day-to-day functioning of individuals' work and social or home environments. Their over-sensitivity in our sample is mainly associated with vestibular and visual stimuli, whereas withdrawal from stimuli is more strongly associated with tactile and vestibular stimuli. Through the analysis we found a statistically significant difference in the presence and degree of sensory sensitization and avoidance of stimuli ($p = 0.0001$). Based on the statistical significance, we confirmed that persons with FMS in our sample had a statistically significant higher presence and degree of sensory hypersensitivity compared to the group of persons without FMS. In the following, we compared the subjective assessment of health-related quality of life indicators in subjects with FMS compared with those in persons without FMS. The indicators were covered under three sub-categories of SF-36 relating to physical health, mental health and social functioning. We also found that there were statistically significant differences between the groups in all three subscales of health-related quality of life ($p < 0.001$). It is evident that individuals without FMS achieved higher results, thereby achieving a better quality of daily life than individuals with FMS in the test group.

The findings broaden our understanding of the important starting points in the relationship between health-related quality of life indicators and their negative effects on day-to-day functioning in patients with FMS with associated sensory modulation disorders, with significant discrepancies across all three sublevels compared with non-FMS subjects.

Regarding the many findings on the significant impact of FMS itself on the psychophysical aspects of patient health, emotional health in such disorders should not be neglected, as many researchers attach a fundamental importance to the regulation of other quality of life indicators (Walston et al. 2006, 991-9). Namely, pain and stress are strongly related phenomena; pain is an activator of the stress and emotional response, and on the other hand, the stress response has a profound effect on perception of pain (O'Conor et al. 2000, 329-31). Hunt et al. (2002, 649-59) identify the two most common mental illnesses that commonly occur with comorbidity, namely depression and anxiety disorders. Liss et al. (2005, 1429-39) found a positive association between SID and the presence of depression and/or anxiety. However, in contrast, the authors Neal et al. (2002, 361-74) found symptoms of sensory disorder only in individuals with anxiety disorder and not with depression. The nature of the relationship between quality of life and FMS with associated SID is therefore quite clear, as many studies already provide good insights into the factors that determine the primary goal of comprehensive treatment of patients with FMS (Bennett 2005, 154-60; Wilbarger and Cook 2011, 653-5). In their study examining the impact of FMS on the well-being of patients with the aforementioned syndrome (n = 27), Walbarger and Cook (2011, 653-6) found a statistically significant positive association in higher stress experience compared to a healthy population (n = 28) in day-to-day life on the side of FMS patients as a result of disturbances in sensory modulation. The degree of psychophysical impairment through the study of pain threshold levels and their impact on quality of life was also found by Marques et al. (2005, 267-70) in a study involving 178 women divided into FMS patients and healthy controls and also came to the same conclusion, with positive correlations in the investigated group. Bernard et al. (2000, 42-9) found in a study of 270 patients with FMS that the psychophysical component of patients' quality of life was statistically significantly related to the intensity and perception of pain, fatigue, depression, cognitive impairment, and perception of the sensation of many sensory stimuli in work and social environments. The review and analysis of numerous scientific studies on the impact of fibromyalgia on the quality of life of patients have also been confirmed by the Mendoza Battle et al. (2014, 4-11), comparing different groups of patients with various rheumatic diseases, including fibromyalgia.

The literature review elicited further relevance of interoperability and extra-perception at lower levels of estimated quality of life by persons with SID. In addition to general disorders in sensory processing, the inclusion of a wider range of specific sensory modalities would also be useful in establishing the correlation between elements of sensory perception and cognitive function, as well as their direct links to mental and physical health (Khalsa 2018, 502-8). Namely, disturbances in sensory processing through external and internal perception can lead to disturbances in cognitive processes, ranging from more intrinsic (learning, memory, evaluation) to extrinsic (attention and concentration), which means that interoceptive information processing can affect all levels of cognition, which again can contribute to many manifestations of mental and physical health disorders (Seth et al. 2011, 395; Khalsa et al. 2018; 501-13). Interoception affects several areas and is associated with all sensory systems, including affective processing of stimuli. Authors Wiens et al. (2000, 417-27) examined this relationship in a healthy population by establishing a relationship between heart rate and experiencing different feelings in persons with disorders in the field of interoceptive information processing. They found a positive association between feeling intensity and heart rate, which again provides a direct correlation between physical and emotional health and modulation disorders in SID. In contrast to interoception, which involves the perception of internal stimuli coming from the body, exteroception refers to how an individual processes external information about the physical world (Quadt et al. 2018, 113-9). It consists of four categories, ranging from the proximal to the distal segments: the somatic sense (tactile system), the chemical senses (olfactory and gustatory system), vision (visual system), and hearing (auditory system). The somatic sense in the tactile system has four major modalities, each mediated through different receptors and neural pathways (Bundy et al. 2002, 40-2; Brietzke et al. 2019; 5-8). The first modality is mechanosensation or discriminatory touch, which allows us to sense the size, shape and texture of objects, as well as to feel their movement across the skin. Proprioception uses somatic feedback from the joints and muscles, which it combines with the information of the vestibular system to represent the perception of the position of the body in space. The third modality relates to signalling in the event of tissue damage or chemical irritation, which is usually perceived as pain or itching, and the fourth represents thermosensation, namely the feeling of heat and cold (Quadt et al. 2018, 112-28; Bundy et al. 2002; 40-2). Numerous studies, including ours, have found positive correlations precisely in sensory dysfunction and symptomatology of FMS, since in most people pain and hypersensitivity are prevalent in symptomatology, which in this case may be due to modulation disorders (Brietzke et al. 2019, 1-9). Coupled with other categories of modulation disorders that are also common in FMS, a marked negative interaction with social, health, and mental quality of life indicators, as well as with cognitive processes in these patients, is expected to be observed. All these factors thus become very important when it comes to patients' capacity for optimal day-to-day functioning (Baranek et al. 2013, 307-20).

So, with the contemporary assumptions of many authors, including Miller et al. (2009; 22), that SID results from the consequent central and peripheral nervous system dysfunction, resulting in increased sensitivity to somatic stimuli, and partly to non-somatic stimuli, research in this area is taking on a whole new dimension. However, studies to find a direct correlation between these indicators are not very large in scope. Therefore, further research will be needed to understand new insights into the pathophysiological mechanism of fibromyalgia and the presence and role of altered sensory processing in this patient population. Of particular importance are the modulating disorders in FMS, which could be the primary cause of the lower threshold for pain perception and increased sensitivity to the adverse effects of exposure to sensory stimuli (Cook et al. 2004, 364-5; Kosek et al. 1996, 375-81; Zimmer and Desch 2012, 1186-9).

Namely, a review of the findings to date shows that some studies confirm the association between changes in the anatomical, chemical, and physiological characteristics of the central nervous system in patients with FMS and their symptomatology. It is found an important psychophysiological aspect that patients with FMS perceive pain and other unpleasant stimuli differently than in healthy subjects, and that normal pain modulating systems such as diffuse inhibitory control mechanisms are impaired in FMS (Schmidt-Wilcke 2007, 110-5). Functional brain imaging studies have demonstrated enhanced activation of the pain system, thereby confirming the reporting of patients with FMS (Gracely et al. 2002, 1333-43; Williams and Gracely 2006, 224; Schmidt-Wilcke 2007, 109-16 Baraniuk et al. 2004, 48). Studies on neurotransmitters have found that abnormalities in the functioning of the dopaminergic, opioid, and serotonergic system have been observed in said patient population (Holman and Myers 2005, 2495-505; Clauw and Crafford 2003, 685-701; Gracely et al. 2002, 1333-43; Williams and Gracely 2006, 224; Yunus and Aldag 1996, 1339; Malt et al. 2003, 77-82; Chudler and Dong 1995, 3-38; Baraniuk et al. 2004, 48; Wik et al. 2003, 619-21; Wik et al. 2006, 1-8; Martikainen et al. 2007, 21-31). Research on the anatomical features of the brain shows structural differences between the brains of FMS patients and the brains of healthy subjects. These changes again provide a compelling explanation for the many signs and symptoms of FMS (Gracely et al. 2002, 1333-43; Cook et al. 2004, 364-78; Zaletel 2010; 47-51). The frequent comorbidity of FMS with stress-related disorders such as chronic fatigue, post-traumatic stress disorder, irritable bowel syndrome, and depression, and the similarity of many central nervous system abnormalities to those of FMS indicate that there is at least partial commonality substrate (Schmidt-Wilcke 2007, 110-5). Today, the diagnosis of fibromyalgia is still based on the subjective reporting of diffuse pain and sensitivity to somatic stimuli, but over the years more pathophysiological abnormalities have been identified. Current research suggests that a change in central nervous system physiology may also be the basis for fibromyalgia symptomatology. All this could lead to completely new perspectives on the etiology of fibromyalgia.

The nature of these changes encourages thinking that people with FMS only report higher levels of pain, or are only hypersensitive to intrinsic and extrinsic stimuli. In doing so, it supports the view that fibromyalgia could be a primary brain disease, or that any changes in the brain are due to a physiological change outside the brain. Central nervous system findings support but do not confirm the view that modulation systems are defective in FMS. This results in an imbalance between facilitation and inhibition, which increases the processing of extrinsic and intrinsic stimuli, which in turn contributes to a greater perception of pain and other sensory stimuli. Similarly, emotional processing of unpleasant and pleasant stimuli can be altered. For this reason, changes in the central nervous system offer a convincing explanation of the main symptoms of FMS, such as pain and emotional response.

However, notwithstanding many contemporary findings, we cannot claim that FMS is a primary brain disorder, since changes in the brain do not necessarily occur at the beginning of the sequence of events leading to the aforementioned condition, wherefore we believe it would be essential to disseminate such research findings.

Through the findings of our study and through the review of numerous other findings that identify a positive correlation of sensory integration dysfunction, accompanying symptoms of fibromyalgia, and higher levels of pain perception in FMS patients, the question of the best options for improving their quality of life through sensory integration therapies raises the comprehensive treatment program. We believe that with this breadth of research into FMS, we can gain insight into the conditions necessary for reducing the symptoms of the syndrome and better managing of the disease, while encouraging at the same time to design and optimize a new model of multidimensional FMS treatment, which is still more difficult to manage.

REFERENCES

[1] Ayres, Anne Jean. 1966. Interrelation of perception, function and treatment. *Journal of the American Physical Therapy Association* 46:741–744.

[2] Ayres, Anne Jean, Zoe Mailloux, and Cathy L. W. Wendler. 1987. Developmental apraxia: Is it a unitary function? *Occupational Therapy Journal of Research* 7(2):93–110.

[3] Ayres, Anne Jean. 2005. *Sensory integration and the child: understanding hidden sensory challenges.* Los Angeles: Western Psychological services.

[4] Baranek, Grace. T., Linda R. Watson, Brian A. Boyd, Michele D. Poe, Fabian J. David, and Lorin McGuire. 2013. Hyperesponsiveness to social and nonsocial sensory stimuli in children with autism, children with developmental delays and tyoically developing children. *Dev Psychopathol* 25(2):307–320.

[5] Baraniuk, James N., Gail Whalen, Jill Cunningham, and Daniel J. Clauw. 2004. Cerebrospinal fluid levels of opioid peptides in fibromyalgia and chronic low back pain. *BMC Musculoskelet Disord* 5:48.

[6] Bennett, Robert. 1981. Fibrositis: misnomer for a common rheumatic disorder. *West J Med* 134:405-413.

[7] Bennett, Robert. 2005. The Fibromyalgia Impact Questionnaire (FIQ): a review of its development, current version, operating characteristics and uses. *Clin Exp Rheumatol* 23(39):154-162.

[8] Bernard, Amy L., Alice Prince, and Patricia Edsall. Quality of Life Issues for Fibromyalgia Patients. 2000. *Arthritis Care and Research* 13(1):42-50.

[9] Blumenstiel, Klaus, Andreas Gerhardt, Roman Rolke, Christiane Bieber, Jonas Tesarz, Hans Christoph Friederich, Wolfgang Eich, and Rolf Detlef Treede. 2011. Quantitative Sensory Testing Profiles in Chronic Back Pain Are Distinct From Those in Fibromyalgia. *The Clinical Journal of Pain* 27(8):682-690.

[10] Brietzke, Aline Patricia, Luciana Conceicao Antunes, Fabiana Carvalho, Jessica Elkifury, Assunta Gasparin, Paulo Roberto Stefani Sanches, Danton Pereira da Silva Junior, Jairo Alberto Dussán-Sarria, Andressa Souza, Iraci Lucena da Silva Torres, Felipe Fregni, and Wolnei Caumo. 2019. Potency of descending pain modulatoy system is linked with peripheral sensory dysfunction in fibromyalgia. *Medicine* 98(3):1-9.

[11] Bundy, Anita C., Shelly J. Lane, and Elisabeth A. Murray. 2002. *Sensory integration: Theory and practice.* 2nd edition. Philadelphia: F.A. Davis Company.

[12] Buskila, D., Neumann L., Sibirski D., and Shvartzman P. 1997. Awareness of diagnostic and clinical features of fibromyalgia among family physicians. *Farm Pract* 14:238-241.

[13] Carrillo-de-la-Peña, Maria Teresa, Miguel Vallet, Royo-Villanova Pérez M. I., and Claudio Gómez Perretta. 2006. Intensity dependence of auditory - evoked cortical potentials in fibromyalgia patients: a test of the generalized hypervigilance hypothesis. *J Pain* 7:480–487.

[14] Chaitow, Leon. 2003. *Fibromyalgia syndrome. A practitioner's guide to treatment.* 2nd edition. London: Churchill Livingstone.

[15] Chudler, Eric H., and Wen-Kui Dong. 1995. The role of the basal ganglia in nociception and pain. *Pain* 60:3-38.

[16] Clauw, Daniel J., and Leslie J. Crofford. 2003. Chronic widespread pain and fibromyalgia: what we know, and what we need to know. *Best Pract Res Clin Rheumatol* 17:685-701.

[17] Cook, Dane B., Gustav Lange, Donald S. Ciccone, Woon Chia Liu, Jason Steffener, and Benjamin H. Natelson. 2004. Functional imaging of pain in patients with primary fibromyalgia. *J Rheumatol* 31:364–378.

[18] Dixon, Eric A., Grant Benham, John A. Sturgeon, Sean Mackey, Kevin A. Johnson, and Jarred Younger. 2016. Development of the Sensory Hypersensitivity Scale (SHS): a self-report tool for assessing sensitivity to sensory stimuli. *J Behav Med* 39(3):537-550.

[19] Dunn, Winnie. 1999. *Sensory Profile user's manual.* San Antonio TX: Psychological Corporation.

[20] Dunn, Winnie, and Catana Brown. 2002. *Adolescent/Adult Sensory Profile*. San Antonio TX: Psychological Corporation.
[21] Geisser, Michael E., Jennifer M. Glass, Ljubinka D. Rajcevska, Daniel J. Clauw, David A. Williams, Paul R. Kileny, and Richard H. Gracely. 2008. A psychophysical study of auditory and pressure sensitivity in patients with fibromyalgia and healthy controls. *J Pain* 9:417–422.
[22] Goldenberg, Don L., Carol Burckhardt, and Leslie Crofford. 2004. Management of Fibromyalgia Syndrome. *JAMA American Medical Association* 292(19):2388-2395.
[23] Gracely, Richard H., Frank Petzke, Julie M. Wolf, and Daniel J. Clauw. 2002. Functional magnetic resonance imaging evidence of augmented pain processing in fibromyalgia. *Arthritis Rheum* 46:1333–1343.
[24] Holman, Andrew J., and Robert R. Myers. 2005. A randomized, doubleblind, placebocontrolled trial of pramipexole, a dopamine agonist, in patients with fibromyalgia receiving concomitant medications. *Arthritis Rheum* 52:2495-505.
[25] Hunt, Caroline, Cath IssaKidis, and Gavin Andrews. 2002. DSM-IV Generalized Auxiety Disorder in the Australian National Survey of Mental Health and Well-Being. *Pshychol Med* 32(4):649-659.
[26] Khalsa, Sahib S., Ralph Adolphs, Oliver G. Cameron, Hugo D. Critchley, Paul W. Davenport, Justin S. Feinstein, Jamie D. Feusner, Sarah N. Garfinkel, Richard D. Lane, Wolf E. Mehling, Alicia E. Meuret, Charles B. Nemeroff, Stephen Oppenheimer, Frederike H. Petzschner, Olga Pollatos, Jamie L. Rhudy, Lawrence P. Schramm, Kyle W. Simmons, Murray B. Stein, Klaas E. Stephan, Omer Van den Bergh, Ilse Van Diest, Andreas von Leupoldt, and Martin P. Paulus. 2018. Interoception and Mental Health: A roadmap. *Bio Pshychiatry Cogn Neurosci Neuroimaging* 3(6):501-5013.
[27] Kosek, Eva, Jan Ekholm, and Per Hansson. 1996. Sensory dysfunction in fibromyalgia patients with implications for pathogenic mechanism. *Pain* 68(2-3):375-383.

[28] Liss, Miriam, Laura Timmel, Kelin Baxley, and Patrick Kilingworth. 2005. Sensory Processing Sensitivity and it's Relation to Pariental Bonding, Anxiety and Depression. *Pers Individ Dif* 39:1429-1439.

[29] Maese, Philip. 2005. Fibromyalgia syndrome: review of clinical presentation, pathogenesis, outcome measures and treatment. *J Rheum Supplements* 75:6-21.

[30] Malt, Eva Albertsen, Snorri Olafsson, Asbjoern Aakvaag, Anders Lund, and Holger Ursin. 2003. Altered dopamine D2 receptor function in fibromyalgia patients: a neuroendocrine study with buspirone in women with fibromyalgia compared to female population based controls. *J Affect Disord* 75:77-82.

[31] Marques, Amélia Pasqual, Elizabeth A.G. Ferreira, Luciana Akemi Matsutani, Carlos Alberto de Bragança Pereira, and Ana Assumpcao. 2005. Quantifying pain threshold and quality of life of fibromalgia patients. *Clin Rheumatol* 24(3):266-271.

[32] Martikainen, Ilkka K., Jussi Hirvonen, Jaana Kajander, Nora Hagelberg, Heikki Mansikka, and Kjell Nagren. 2007. Correlation of human cold pressor pain responses with 5-HT(1A) receptor binding in the brain. *Brain Res* 1172:21-31.

[33] Maruish, Mark E. 2011. *User's manual for the SF-36v2*. Lincoln, RI, USA: Quality Metric Incorporated.

[34] McIntosh, Daniel N., Lucy Jane Miller, Vivian Shyu, and Randi J. Hagerman. 1999. Sensory-modulation disruption, electrodermal responses, and functional behaviors. *Dev Med Child Neurol* 41:608–615.

[35] Mendoza Battle, Florina, Regina Okun, and Ashlee Sand. 2014. The Impact of Fibromyalgia and Sensory Processing on Participation of Daily Activities. *Master's Theses and Capstone Projects*. 14. Accessed February 14, 2020. https://scholar.dominican.edu/masters-theses/14.

[36] Miller, Lucy Jane, Marie E. Anzalone, Shelly J. Lane, Sharon A. Cermak, and Elizabeth T. Osten. 2007. Concept Evolution in Sensory Integration: A Proposed Nosology for Diagnosis. *Am J Occup Ther* 61(2):135-140.

[37] Miller, Lucy Jane, Darci M. Nielsen, Sarah A. Schoen, and Barbara A. Brett-Green. 2009. Perspectives on Sensory Processing Disorder: a Call for Translational Research. *Front Integr Neurosci* 3:22.

[38] Miller, Lucy Jane, Sarah A. Schoen, Shelly Mulligan, and Jillian Sullivan. 2017. Identification of Sensory Processing and Integration Symptom Clusters: A Preliminary Study. *Occupational Therapy International.* Accessed January 16, 2020. Doi:10.1155/2017/2876080.

[39] Montoya, Pedro José, Carolina Sitges, Manuel García-Herrera, Raúl Izquierdo, Magdalena Truyols, Nicole Blay, and Dolores Less Collado. 2006. Reduced brain habituation to somatosensory stimulation in patients with fibromyalgia. *Arthritis Rheum* 54:1995–2003.

[40] Neal, Jo Anne, Robert J. Edelmann, and Martin Glachan. 2002. Behavioral Inhibition and Symptoms of Anxiety and Depression: Is there a Specific Relationship with Social Phobia? *Br J Clin Psychol* 41(4):361-74.

[41] O'Conor, T. M., O'Halloran D. J., Shanahan F. 2000. The Stress Response and the Hypothalamic-Pituitary - Adrenal Axis: From Molecule to Melancholia. *Q J Med* 93:323-333.

[42] Pearson Education. 2008. *Technical Report: Adolescent/Adult Sensory Profile. Sensory Profile School Companion (SPSC).* Accessed March 18, 2020. www.SensoryProfile.com.

[43] Quadt, Lisa, Hugo D. Critchley, and Sarah N. Garfinkel. 2018. The Neurobiology of Interoception in Health and Disease. *Ann NY Acad Sci* 1428(1):112-128.

[44] Salaffi, Fausto, Piercarlo Sarzi Puttini, Rita Girolimetti, Fabiola Atzeni, Stefania Gasparini, and Walter Grassi. 2009. Health-related quality of life in fibromyalgia patients: a comparison with rheumatoid arthritis patients and the general population using the SF-36 health survey. *Clin Exp Rheumatol* 27(56):67-74.

[45] Schaaf, Rosseann, and Zoe Mailloux. 2015. *Clinican's quide for implementig Ayres sensory integration: Promoting participation for*

children with autism. Bethesda: The American Occupational Therapy Association, Inc.

[46] Schmidt-Wilcke, Tobias, Luerding Ralf, Weigand Teresa, Jurgens Tim, Schuierer Gerhard, and Leinisch Elke. 2007. Striatal grey matter increase in patients suffering from fibromyalgia - a voxel-based morphometry study. *Pain* 132(1):109-16.

[47] Schoen, Sarah A., Lucy J. Miller, and Julian C. Sullivan. 2014. Measurment in Sensory Modulation: The Sensory Processing Scale Assessment. *Am J Occup Ther* 68(5):522-530.

[48] Schwartz, Benett L., and John. H. Krantz. 2019. *Sensation and Perception.* 2nd edition. USA: SAGE Publications, Inc.

[49] Seth, Anil K., Keisuke Suzuki, and Hugo D. Critchley. 2011. An Interoceptive Predictive Coding Model of Conscious Presence. *Front Pshychol* 2:395.

[50] Smith Roley, Sussanne, Zoe Mailloux, Heather Miller-Kuhaneck, and Tara J. Glennon. 2007. Understanding Ayres' Sensory Integration. *OT Practice* 12(7).

[51] Smith, Bruce W., Erin M. Tooley, Erica Q. Montaque, Amanda E. Robinson, Cynthia J. Cosper, and Paul G. Mullins. 2008. Habituation and sensitization to heat and cold pain in women with fibromyalgia and healthy controls. *Pain* 140(3):420-428.

[52] Smythe, Hugh A., and Harvey Moldofsky. 1977. Two contributions to understanding of the "fibrositis" syndrome. *Bull Rheum Dis* 28:928-931.

[53] Ubago Linares, Ma del Carmen, Isabel Ruiz-Perez, Ma Jose Bermejo Perez, Antonio Olry de Labry-Lima, Elisa Hernandez-Torres, and Juncal Plazaola-Castano. 2008. Analysis of the impact of fibromyalgia on quality of life: associated factors. *Clin Rheumatol* 27(5):613-619.

[54] Walston, Jeremy, Evan C. Hadley, Luigi Ferrucci, Jack M. Guralnik, Anne B. Newman, Stephanie A. Studenski. 2006. Research Agenda for Frailty in Older Adults: toward a Better Undarstanding of Physiology and Etiology. *J Am Geriatr Soc* 54:991-1001.

[55] Wiens, Stefan, Elizabeth S. Mezzacappa, and Edward S. Katkin. 2000. Hearthbeat Detection and the Experience of Emotion. *Cogn Emot* 14:417-427.
[56] Wik, G., Fischer H., Bragee B., Kristianson M., and Fredrikson M. 2003. Retrosplenial cortical activation in the fibromyalgia syndrome. *Neuro Report* 14:619-621.
[57] Wik, G., Fischer H., Finer B., Bragee B., Kristianson M., and Fredrikson M. 2006. Retrospenial cortical deactivation during painful stimulation of fibromyalgic patients. *Int J Neurosci* 116:1-8.
[58] Wilbarger, Julia L., and Dane B. Cook. 2011. Multisensory Hypersensitivity in Women With Fibromyalgia: Implications for Well Being and Intervention. *Arch Phys Med Rehabil* 92(4):653-6.
[59] Williams, David A., and Richard H. Gracely. 2006. Biology and therapy of fibromyalgia. Functional magnetic resonance imaging findings in fibromyalgia. *Arthritis Res Ther* 8:224.
[60] Wolfe, Frederick. 1986. Development of criteria for the diagnosis of fibrositis. *Am J Med* 81:99-104.
[61] Wolfe, Frederick, Smythe A. Hugh, Muhammad B. Yunus, Robert M. Bennett, Claire Bombardier, Don L. Goldenberg, Peter Tugwell, Stephen M. Campbell, Micha Abeles, Patricia Clark, Adel G. Fam, Stephen J. Farber, Justus J. Fiechtner, C. Michael Franklin, Robert A. Gatter, Daniel Hamaty, James Lessard, Alan. S. LichtBroun, Alfonse T. Masi, Glenn A. McCain, John W. Reynolds, Thomas J. Romano, Jon I. Russel, and Robert P. Sheon. 1990. The American College of Rheumatology 1990 Criteria for the Classification of Fibromyalgia. *Arth and Rheum* 33(2):160-172.
[62] Wolfe, Frederick, Daniel J. Clauw, Mary-Ann Fitzgharles, Don L. Goldenberg, Robert S. Katz, Philip Mease, Anthony S. Russell, Jon I. Russell, John B. Winfield, and Muhammad B. Yunus. 2010. The American College of Rheumatology Preliminary Diagnostic Criteria for Fibromyalgia and Measurment of Symptom Severity. *Arthritis Care and Research* 62(5):600-610.
[63] Yunus, Muhammad B., Alfonse T. Masi, John J. Calabro, Kenneth A. Miller, and Seth L. Feigenbaum. 1981. Primary fibromyalgia

(fibrositis): clinical study of 50 patients with matched normal controls. *Semin Arth Rheum* 11:151-171.

[64] Yunus, Muhammad B., Alfonse T. Masi, and Jean C. Aldag. 1989. Preliminary criteria for primary fibromyalgia syndrome (PFS): multivariate analysis of a consecutive series of PHS, other pain patients, and normaln subjects. *Clin Exp Rheumatol* 7:63-69.

[65] Yunus, Muhammad B., and Jean C. Aldag. 1996. Restless legs syndrome and leg cramps in fibromyalgia syndrome: a controlled study. *BMJ* 312:1339.

[66] Yunus, Muhammad B., and Jean C. Aldag. 2012. The concept of incomplete fibromyalgia syndrome: comparison of incomplete fibromyalgia syndrome with fibromyalgia syndrome by 1990 ACR classification criteria and its implications for newer criteria and clinical practice. *J Clin Rheumatol* 18:71-75.

[67] Zaletel, Marjan. Treatment of Fibromyalgia. 2010. *Rehabilitation* 9(2):47-52.

[68] Zimmer, Michelle, and Larry Desch. 2012. Sensory Integration Therapies for Children with Developmental and Behavioral Disorders. *Pediatrics* 129(6):1186-1187.

In: Medical Care
Editor: Brian A. Soileau

ISBN: 978-1-53618-048-0
© 2020 Nova Science Publishers, Inc.

Chapter 2

THE IMPORTANCE FOR IMPROVEMENT OF THE EXISTING GMFM SCORE IN NEUROLOGICAL DISORDERS

Alen Kapel[1], Tine Kovacic[1], Natasa Kos[1,2] and Tomaz Velnar[1,3,]*

[1]Alma Mater Europaea-ECM Maribor, Maribor, Slovenia
[2]Department of Rehabilitational Medicine,
University Medical Centre Ljubljana,
Ljubljana, Slovenia
[3]Department of Neurosurgery,
University Medical Centre Ljubljana,
Ljubljana, Slovenia

ABSTRACT

Despite many various scores and ways of assessment that have been developed so far for the evaluation of motor functions in persons with special needs, there is still no perfect score existing. Gross Motor

---

* Corresponding Author's Email: tvelnar@hotmail.com.

Function Measure is a useful scale for evaluating the gross motor function of persons with special needs. There are two versions of the GMFM in use, the 66 and 88. They differ in the types of disorders being used for. In this study, we propose an improved version of the GMFM score, including movement quality, quality of locomotor execution and postural characteristics. An improved version of the GMFM was tested by neurophysiotherapists in five girls with Rett syndrome. The improved version was also examined by 49 neurophysotherapist and 19 doctors. Although the GMFM-88 provides key factors in subject's gross motor function status, it is not able to provide or evaluate the quality of motor ability concerning movement, execution and transition quality, multidimensional movement and postural characteristics in sitting and standing position. The results confirmed that the modified GMFM-88, including all these parameters, was a valid and reliable instrument for evaluating gross motor function for a specific group of neurological disorders. These new elements are thus essential factors added in the modified GMFM and form a part of a more thorough multidisciplinary interventional approach in the treatment of Rett syndrome patients.

Keywords: Rett syndrome, neurological disorders, gross motor function, GMFM score, modified GMFM score

INTRODUCTION

Neurological disorders are diseases affecting the central and peripheral nervous system which result in various impairments. One of the rarest neurological disorders is the Rett syndrome (RS), also known as a progressive neurodevelopmental disorder appearing almost exclusively in girls and causing severe defects, which affect the ability to speak, move, feed and breathe [1, 2]. According to the data obtained by the neurological department of the paediatric clinic of the University Medical Centre Ljubljana, there were 18 girls diagnosed with RS in Slovenia in 2020.

Diagnostic protocols are based on main and supportive criteria. In RS this criteria includes clinical features of loss or decreased manual skills, reduction or loss of speech, stereotypical arm movements, decreased or loss of communication skills, microcephaly and regressed social interaction with subsequent improvement, breathing disorders (hyperventilation and holding of breath) in conscious state, swallowing air and abdominal tension, bruxism, incorrect spatial movement, altered sleeping patterns, unjustified screaming and laughing, cold and blue feet, sensory reduction to pain and presence of kyphosis and scoliosis [3].

The purpose of the study was to demonstrate the developmental complexity of RS, present insufficiencies of the GMFM-88 score, introduce the modified GMFM-88 score and practically research the level of usefulness of the GMFM-88 and the modified GMFM-88 scores among neurophysiotherapists and doctors. The goal of the study was to introduce the GMFM-88 score that was improved with parameters and to show its usefulness in multidisciplinary habilitation.

Medical Scores

Medical scores are evaluation tools to determine clinical decisions, decision-making and clinical management [4]. They evaluate patient's condition and also enable monitoring of their improvement in treatment. Although scores are used in different fields of medicine and are carried out by different types of medical professionals, they are nonetheless important for scoring systems to be based on easily recordable variables, they should be well calibrated, have a high level of discrimination, should be applicable to all patient populations, could be used internationally and be able to predict a functional status or quality of life [5].

A Romanian study has shown that scores in emergency medicine and other areas of intensive medicine, as well as in patient management procedures, are becoming increasingly efficient [4].

Although many different scores exist, GMFM is a reliable, valid and useful score for evaluating and detecting gross motor function and development of persons with neurological disorders [6]. The score is commonly used for clinical and research purposes [5, 6]. Two versions of the GMFM scale are in use, the 66 and the 88. They differ in calculated scores and suitability. The 66 version calculates scores only as a total, and is therefore not suitable for infants, whereas the 88 version splits evaluation scores in five dimensions [6]. Some studies have shown that the GMFM-88 provides only minor progression or regression results in children with neurological disorders. Other studies also attest for GMFM-88 to be used to monitor activity focused interventions [6, 7]. It was found that GMFM-88 should be used in children with low motor capability and the 66 version in children with advanced motor capability [6].

When evaluating the gross motor function in girls with RS, we used the Gross Motor Function Measure 88 score (GMFM-88). It determines the ability to perform particular motor skill and allows to set the condition of gross motor function and assess progress of habilitation with regards to gross motor function.

Clinical Features

Prenatal, perinatal and postnatal periods in girls are normal, although some studies show motor and behaviour anomalies, hypotonia and issues with feeding between 6 to 18 months of age [8-11]. Motor skills are generally weakened, only stereotypical arm movements can be recognised [12, 13]. At that age, it is difficult to speak of RS, since these pathologies are hard to detect [9, 14, 15]. Stagnation development phase extends from 6 to 18 months of age. Psychomotor development slows down and the body becomes hypotonic [8, 9, 14]. Regression phase occurs between the ages 1 and 4 and involves aphasia and regression of arm control [8, 9, 14]. Ataxia and apraxia appear in the transition period between the second and third phase [8]. The third phase, called plateau period, occurs between the ages 4 and 7 and involves a reduction of autistic behaviour, improved use of arms, a decrease in gross motor function and other motor and cognitive functions [1, 2]. The final development phase of RS occurs between the ages 5 and 15 and is called the phase of late motor deterioration. Gross motor function deteriorates with age, hypotonicity progresses into hypertonicity and rigidity [1, 8]. More than 80% of girls suffer from dystonia and progressive scoliosis, most also from muscular asymmetry, deformities of lower extremities and balance disorders which cause motor impairment and subsequent loss on mobility and development of osteopenia [1, 3, 8]. More than 97% of RS cases can be distinguished between them, which makes it difficult to create a basic diagnostics model for RS, one that would serve during potential diagnostics [9, 11, 13].

DATA AND METHODS

The study addressed the complexity of RS, significance of regular assessments of the gross motor function in persons diagnosed with RS by using the GMFM-88 score, introduction of the modified GMFM-88 score and neurophysiotherapists' and doctors' perspectives on the use of the general and the modified GMFM-88 scores in practice and in an interdisciplinary and multidisciplinary habilitation team.

We have used GMFM-88 for assessing the gross motor function in girls with RS and a modified score GMFM-88, where we added parameters related to the quality of motor skills concerning movement, execution and transition quality, multidimensional movement and postural characteristics in sitting and standing positions and social interaction.

The GMFM-88 gross motor function score is reliable, relevant and responsive, and due to its specifics, it has been approved for evaluation of persons with RS.

The first part of the study included five girls diagnosed with RS and four neurophysiotherapists with specific expertise in neurodevelopmental therapy, who determined the girls' condition of gross motor function based on the GMFM-88 and the modified GMFM-88 scores. Girls were selected randomly, according to the probability type sampling. All five girls and the four neurophysiotherapists come from one of the social institutions in Slovenia.

The other part of the research involved 49 neurophysiotherapists and 19 doctors from the field of physiotherapy and paediatrics, who participated in a questionnaire with 9 closed-type questions in relation to the GMFM-88 and the modified GMFM-88 score.

Data was statistically processed using the SPSS software (Statistical Package for the Social Sciences 21). We used tabulation for presentation of quantitative data. The study was carried out in accordance with the principles of International Code of Medical Ethics and the Helsinki/Tokyo Declaration. We have obtained the consensus from the Commission of the Republic of Slovenia for medical ethics (no. 0120-47/2018/4), and consensus of the Scientific Council of the Social and Security Institution which the patients are part of.

Questionnaire regarding GMFM-88 and modified GMFM-88

Question 1 – Is GMFM-88 time efficiant?
Question 2 – Do you consider GMFM-88 as a limited score regarding evaluation status?
Question 3 – GMFM-88 results are relevant only for medical and neurophysiotherapy professionals?
Question 4 – Is GMFM-88 a thorough score in a multidisciplinary habilitation intervention?
Question 5 – Does the modified GMFM-88 provides needed evaluation parameters for an interdisciplinary intervention?
Question 6 – Does the modified GMFM-88 provides needed evaluation parameters for a multidisciplinary intervention?
Question 7 – Is social interaction monitoring important in habilitation of girls with Rett syndrome?
Question 8 – Should there be a modified GMFM-88 for a multidisciplinary approach?
Question 9 – Is the Modified GMFM-88 time efficiant?

RESULTS

Firstly, this study demonstrated the differences between the GMFM-88 and the modified version of GMFM-88 score with the inclusion of five girls with diagnosed RS, who were evaluated by four neurophysiotherapists using the GMFM-88 and the modified GMFM-88 scores for determining their condition. The ages of participating girls were 18, 26, 28, 28 and 45 with the mean age of 29 and all of the participating neurophysiotherapists were specialised in neurodevelopmental therapy. Secondly, this study provides medical and neurophysiotherapeutic professional opinion on the GMFM-88 and the modified version of GMFM-88 scores. 49 neurophysiotherapists and 19 doctors (paediatricians and physicians) were included in this study. The modified GMFM-88 score includes parameters that show quality of motor ability concerning movement, execution and transition quality, multidimensional movement and postural characteristics in sitting and standing position and social interaction.

Table 1 (GMFM-88) and 2 (modified GMFM-88) provide evaluation results for five girls with RS.

Table 1. Results of the GMFM-88 evaluation

Reference number of girl with RS	Birth year	GMFM-88 Dimension score in %					Total score
		A	B	C	D	E	
1	1993	54.90	85	52.38	61.5	38.88	58.53
2	1991	5.88	8.33	7.14	7.69	6.94	7.19
3	1991	64.70	58.33	4.76	30.77	20.83	35.87
4	1974	54.90	21.67	0.00	2.56	11.11	18.04
5	2001	50.98	35.00	2.38	5.12	6.94	20.08

A: lying and rolling, B: sitting, C: crawling and kneeling, D: standing, E: walking, running, jumping

Table 2. Modified GMFM-88 results

Dimension/no.	Parameter	Reference number of girl with RS				
		1	2	3	4	5
A/1	Spacity or contracture hinders hip flexion	yes	yes	no	no	yes
A/2	Spacity or contracture hinders knee flexion	yes	yes	yes	no	yes
A/3	Turning on flank with assist	no	yes	yes	yes	yes
A/4	Girl is cooperating	yes	yes	yes	yes	yes
A/5	Rise of head is isolated	no	no	no	no	no
B/1	Activity is limited by hipotony	no	yes	no	no	no
B/2	Response on external stimuli	yes	yes	yes	yes	yes
B/3	Intercepted reactions	yes	no	yes	no	no
B/4	Straightening reactions	yes	no	yes	yes	yes
B/5	Equilibrium reactions	no	no	no	no	no
C/1	Realisation limited due contractures or spacity	yes	yes	yes	yes	yes
C/2	Kneeling is possible only assisted	no	yes	no	no	no
E/1	Static balance	yes	no	yes	no	no
E/2	Dinamic balance	no	no	no	no	no

Both evaluations were made by four neurophysiotherapists specialised in neurodevelopmental therapy. The GMFM-88 provides results only by percentage and establishes only in what range the activity was executed, without including other parameters. The modified GMFM-88 score is an updated version of the existing GMFM-88 score and shows parameters for establishing a wide range of insights into causes for inability to start or accomplish GMFM-88 activities. Table 3 demonstrates questionnaire results regarding neurophysiotherapists' and doctors' position on the GMFM-88 and the modified GMFM-88 scores. 80% of neurophysiotherapists and 68.5% of doctors, who participated, determined that the modified GMFM-88 score was necessary to fulfil requirements for a multidisciplinary approach, and that the score brings additional data, relevant for the multidisciplinary approach.

Table 3. Questionnaire results

Question no.	Results				Results in %			
	Neurophysiotherapist		Doctor		Neurophysiotherapist		Doctor	
	Yes	No	Yes	No	Yes	No	Yes	No
1	0	47	0	19	0	100	0	100
2	31	16	8	11	66	34	42	58
3	38	9	19	0	71	19	100	0
4	8	39	14	5	17	83	73.7	26.3
5	29	18	16	3	62	38	66.7	33.3
6	34	13	12	7	72.4	27.6	63	37
7	47	0	16	3	100	0	66.7	33.3
8	38	9	13	6	80	20	68.5	31.5
9	0	47	0	19	0	100	0	100

72.4% of participating neurophysiotherapists and 63% doctors agreed with the latter. The majority of neurophysiotherapists (62%) and doctors (66,7%) determined that GMFM-88 provides the necessary evaluation parameters for an interdisciplinary intervention and the majority of them also determined the modified GMFM-88 as a score for providing parameters for multidisciplinary intervention.

All of them (100% of neurophysiotherapists and 100% of doctors) confirmed that both, the GMFM-88 and the modified GMFM-88 scores are time consuming and that the GMFM-88 was relevant exclusively to medical and neurophysiotherapeutic professionals.

DISCUSSION

The symptomatology in RS is predominately related to mobility disorders and issues, therefore neurophysiotherapeutic treatment is crucial since we wish to use the neurophysiotherapeutic approach to maintain and improve motor skills, develop or maintain the existing ability to transfer, decrease or prevent deformities, ease discomfort or irritability and improve the level of autonomy. Numerous scores can be used to determine the condition and assess progress. RS most significantly affects the gross motor function, therefore, girls with RS are assessed with the GMFM-88 score which evaluates five types of movement - lying and turning, sitting, climbing and kneeling, standing, walking, running and jumping. A clinical challenge appears when identifying phenotypic features of RS, if slurred speech and social deficit are present at an early development phase. The latter can be related to the Australian study which shows that the mean age of the beginning of regression is 18 months, whereas the mean age of diagnosing RS is 33 months [1, 9]. Atypical development is at first diagnosed as autism and only later in regression phase as the RS. In rare cases there is no diagnose given until regression of development appears [11, 16, 17].

Gross motor function plays a role in many aspects of everyday life with its limitations caused by the atypical postural characteristics, righting techniques, fine motor control, coordination, conscious movement and the rest [6-9]. Compared to the normal motor development of a child in the stagnation phase of RS, the child reliably supports itself on palms, with its arms fully extended, turning from back to belly is coordinated, controlled and involves relevant arm and leg movements [8].

The study brings knowledge on developmental complexity of RS and its evaluation and introduction of insufficiencies of the GMFM-88 score by proposing an introduction of an improved, modified GMFM-88 score and by defining the significance of the GMFM-88 and the modified GMFM-88 scores among neurophysiotherapists and doctors. The GMFM-88 gross motor function score is reliable, valid and responsive score for children with cerebral palsy. Due to its specifics it has also been approved for evaluation of persons with RS. In a clinical environment, the GMFM-88 score is often used in particular for evaluation of progress in special treatment. Due to the extent and the duration of evaluation, the procedure must be performed by an experienced professional, since the course of evaluation is physically demanding for the patient, which may lead to incorrect data and thus, to incorrect assessment of condition [3, 6, 9].

The score consists of numeric assessment which includes four phases. However, it does not include parameters related to the quality of executed movement or present external factors. Due to the latter, we have supplemented the score with parameters related to social interaction (grimaces), spasticity and contractures, asymmetrical movement, head control, coordination of manual skill, interaction with a therapist, head control, balance, coordination when turning, influence of external factors, intercepting, righting and balancing function, pelvis control, static and dynamic balance, leg coordination and walk quality.

Using the GMFM-88 gross motor function, we have established that compared to a normally developing child, our girls with RS did not have fully developed functions for lying and turning from back to belly, i.e., the movement in both of these positions was hindered and incomplete. The GMFM-88 score only determines that it was not possible to perform an activity and fails to determine the cause. Using the modified GMFM-88 score, we established that activities were hindered by contractures or spasms in knees or hips and that the head does lift, yet the movements are not isolated and that turning on a hip can be performed only with assistance. Movement also wasn't harmonised with arm and leg coordination. The girls also fail to develop motor coordination that would allow typical crawling and positioning on all fours. With the help of the modified GMFM-88 score, we managed to establish that the execution of activity is limited due to contractures and spasticity, and in individuals who were able to complete activities, the kneeling was only possible with provided assistance.

In the field B, which includes sitting, we established that at the beginning of habilitation, the sitting function was once again limited and that girls were unable to maintain their position, since their righting techniques are atypically developed. Hypotonia of righting musculature in childhood and subsequent hypertonicity in adulthood, are the reason that spasticity usually first occurs in lower extremities. Based on the muscle tone, 30% of grown up females are hypotonic, 40% are spastic and 30%

are dystonic [1-3]. Gradual increase of muscle tone causes an asymmetric reaction in form of lateral torso tilt and subsequent cause of scoliosis and kyphosis [2, 3, 8]. The study which analysed sitting, proves that merely 1/3 of girls were able to independently sit on the floor or in a chair [10]. Compared to the GMFM-88, which found that the girls were unable to maintain their sitting position, the modified GMFM-88 score allowed us to establish that girls with greater success in the field C all possess intercepting, righting and balancing reactions which are limited to maintaining position prior to falling, but do not allow returning to the starting position. We also discovered that all girls responded to external impulses in form of toys and voices but not all reached out for toys. One girl was unable to perform activities due to hypotonicity.

Studies also indicate that one quarter of girls had scoliosis by the age of 6, and three quarters of girls by the age of 13. Girls who experienced difficulties in development in their first 6 months after birth, are more prone to incidence of scoliosis by the age 6 [18].

On average, scoliosis progresses by 14 degrees annually [1, 8, 18], therefore, monitoring of the spine curve is mandatory during the annual examination which could also be included in the modified GMFM-88 score. A severe case of scoliosis is predicted when the scoliosis symptoms appear prior to the age of 5, when girls were already hypotonic in childhood and unable to walk, or were able to walk and later quickly lost the ability. 61% of immobile patients and 25% of mobile patients require surgical correction of scoliosis. Scoliosis and kyphosis appear due to asymmetrical muscular tone [8, 11, 18]. Our research showed that despite the annual regression, the lowest score during assessment of sitting was not achieved by the oldest patient, and similarly, the highest score was not achieved by the youngest participant.

The ability to stand and walk depends on body coordination. 50 to 85% of girls master the ability to walk, some lose this ability later throughout their development, others are never able to walk [4, 8, 19]. The extent of inability among girls varies, some are incapable to independently turn while standing, independently sit and independently transfer from floor to a chair [8, 21].

During inspection of our sample with the GMFM-88 and the modified GMFM-88 scores, we established that all girls depend on assistance. Standing and walking were performed with support, whereas complex motor patterns, such as running and jumping, were not achieved. Only two girls were able to maintain static balance and none of the girls could maintain dynamic balance without additional support. Study which focused on the ability to stand and walk discovered that most of the sample required assistance when standing and walking. 18% of the girls were able to stand and walk independently. Less than 7% could perform complex motor patterns such as sideways marching and a 180° turn. The ability to stand and walk among individuals with rigid and flat feet was low, and high in girls with flexible flat feet. Age and body weight distribution are positively connected when standing [10].

If we compare the latter with typical development, the children usually perform their first independent forward steps in their 12th month. Due to symmetrical distribution of body weight their steps are somewhat wider and the use of arms is based on balancing. Coordination of arm movement is harmonised since the sensorimotor intelligence has already appeared. In the thirteenth month, orientation and spatial coordination are at a higher level. Walking in the centre of a space is possible without support, change of direction of movement is also smoother, while girls with RS in our sample weren't able to achieve complex motor patterns and only 7% of girls in our study which examined walking and standing were able to achieve complex motor patterns.

Healthy developing children use arms to balance themselves when walking, whereas a girl with RS is unable to balance and can only do so while holding onto a fix object on which they put most of their weight. Muscle functioning in typical development is executed based on nerve impulses which determine whether flexion or extension are performed, whilst in persons with RS, the neurological disorder affects the muscle tone resulting in impaired or impossible execution of particular movements [8, 9].

Body symmetry negatively impacts the ability to walk and stand with regards to more difficult weight distribution [10]. With the modified

GMFM-88 score, we established that the biggest issue possessed the dynamic balancing which was not achieved without additional support in form of assistance. Scoliosis deteriorates with age. Inability to correctly distribute weight with feet negatively impacts the ability to walk and stand. The reason for this is not solely scoliosis but in certain cases a shortened hip adductor and flexor which additionally prevent symmetrical weight distribution. Maintaining mobility is significant due to incidence of osteopenia and osteoporosis [8, 22].

It has been proven that a shortened Achilles tendon and posterior pelvis tilt result in the loss of the ability to walk. The reduction of the ability is on the other hand caused by progressive muscle shortenings and joint deformities [8, 9, 18].

Muscle shortening causes joint deformities and additionally impacts the motor function of girls. In most cases, the hip adductor and flexor are shortened [8]. Balanced body weight distribution is impossible in a standing position which causes poor balance and results in inability to independently walk [8]. Standing and walking must be maintained in order to prevent osteopenia and osteoporosis. Decreased bone density is common for RS [18-22].

In normal development, the children usually perform their first independent forward steps in their 12th month, their steps are somewhat wider and they use arms for balancing. Coordination of arm movements is harmonised since the sensorimotor intelligence has already appeared. Orientation and spatial coordination are at a higher level in the thirteenth month [1].

Standing in the centre of a space is achievable without support and changing direction is smoother. Healthy developing children use arms to balance themselves when walking, whereas a girl with RS is unable to balance and can only do so while holding onto a fix object on which they put most of their weight. Muscle functioning in normal development is based on nerve impulses which determine whether flexion or extension are performed, whilst in persons with RS, the neurological disorder affects the muscle tone which results in impaired or impossible execution of particular movements [8, 15].

CONCLUSION

The differences between the modified GMFM-88 score and the GMFM-88 score are mainly in the observance of parameters which potentially prevent execution of certain activities. We established that both, the GMFM-88 and the modified GMFM-88 scores aren't time efficient, but involve a long-term evaluation process which in most cases provides accurate information on the condition of the gross motor function. The modified GMFM-88 score additionally provides results related to reasons for values of individual GMFM-88 chapters. RS habilitation occurs at an interdisciplinary or multidisciplinary level, therefore all of atypical motor patterns must be evaluated and put on record. This presents the only means to show the entire condition of gross motor function used for determining the course of habilitation. The modified GMFM-88 score is the first step in solving the issue of ensuring an adequate evaluation documentation which would allow all interventions to be driven towards activity-related goals, activity-focused intervention and impairment-focused intervention [23, 24]. Data interpretation will be easier within an interdisciplinary or multidisciplinary team, since their reasons will also be known besides the numeric data. The latter will be useful when setting goals not only in their own professional field but will allow them to connect their fields with interventions in the field of gross motor function which is the goal of interdisciplinary and multidisciplinary (re)habilitation.

REFERENCES

[1] Percy, A. K. (2016). Progress in Rett syndrome: from discovery to clinical trials. *Wien Med. Wochenschr.,* 166 (11): 325 - 332. Accessed November 3, 2019. doi: 10.1007/s10354-016-0491-9.

[2] Kyle, M. S., Vashi, N. and Justice, M. J. (2018). Rett syndrome: a neurological disorder with metabolic components. *Open Biol.,* 8 (2): 1 - 17. Accessed November 3, 2019. doi: 10.1098/rsob.170216.

[3] Neul, J. L., Kaufmann, W. E., Glaze, D. G., Christodoulou, J., Clarke, A. J., Buisson, B. N. et al. (2010). Rett syndrome: revised diagnostic criteria and nomenclature. *Ann. Neurol.*, 68 (6): 944 - 950. Accessed November 3, 2019. doi: 10.1002/ana.22124.

[4] Oprita, B., Aignatova, B. and Gabor-Postole, D. A. (2014). Scores and scales used in emergency medicine. *Journal of Medicine and Life,* 7 (3): 4 - 7. Accessed November 3, 2019. doi:25870686.

[5] Keegan, M. T., Gajic, O. and Afessa, B. (2011). Severity of illness scoring systems in the intensive care unit. *Crit. Care Med.*, 39 (1): 163 - 169. Accessed November 3, 2019. doi: 10.1097/CCM.0b013e3181f96f81.

[6] Hielkema, T., Hamer, E. G., Ebbers, I., Dirks, T., Maathuis, C., Reinders, H., Geertzen, J. et al. (2013). GMFM in infancy:Age-specific limitations and adaptations. *Pediatric Physical Therapy*, 25 (2): 168 - 176. Accessed November 3, 2019. doi: 10.1097/PEP.0b013e318288d370.

[7] Kor, J. (2017). Functional improvement after the gross motor function measure-88 item based training in childer with cerebral palsy. *Phys. Ther.*, 29 (3): 115 - 121. Accessed November 3, 2019. doi: 10.18857/jkpt.2017.29.3.115.

[8] Lotan, M., Hanks, S. (2006). Physical therapy intervention for individuals with Rett syndrome. *The Scientific World Journal*, 187 (6): 1314-1338. Accessed November 3, 2019. doi: 10.1100/tsw.2006.187.

[9] Fehr, S., Bebbington, A., Ellaway, C., Rowe, P., Leonard, H. and Downs, J. (2010). Altered attainment of developmental milestones influences the age of diagnosis of Rett syndrome. *J. Child Neurology,* 0 (00): 1 - 8. Accessed November 3, 2019. doi: 10.1177/0883073811401396.

[10] Borst, E. H., Townend, S. G., Eck, M., Smeets, E., Berg, M., Laan, A. and Curfs, G. L. (2018). Abnormal foot position and standing and walking ability in Rett syndrome. *J. Dev. Phys. Disabil.*, 30 (2): 281 - 295. Accessed November 3, 2019. doi: 10.1007/s10882-017-9585-6.

[11] Fehr, S., Downs, J., Bebbington, A. and Leonard, H. (2010). Atypical presentations and specific genotypes are associated with a delay in diagnosis in females with Rett syndrome. *Am. J. Med. Genet. A,* 0 (10): 2535 - 2542. Accessed November 3, 2019. doi: 10.1002/ajmg.a.33640.

[12] Downs, J., Bebbington, A., Jacoby, P., Williams, A. M., Ghosh, S., Kaufmann, W. and Leonard, H. (2010). Level of purposeful hand function as a marker of clinical severity in Rett syndrome. *Dev. Med. Child Neurol.,* 52 (9): 817 - 23. Accessed November 3, 2019. doi: 10.1111/j.1469-8749.2010.03636.x.

[13] Carter, P., Downs, J., Bebbington, A., Williams, S., Jacoby, P., Kaufmann, W. and Leonard, H. (2010). Stereotypical hand movements in 144 subjects with Rett syndrome from the population-based Australian database. *Movement disorders,* 25 (3): 282 - 288. Accessed November 3, 2019. doi: 10.1002/mds.22851.

[14] Downs, J., Stahlhut, M., Wong, K., Sygler, B., Bisgaard, A. M., Jacoby, P. et al. (2016). Validating the Rett syndrome gross motor scale. *PLoS One,* 11 (1): 1 - 11. Accessed November 3, 2019. doi: 10.1371/journal.pone.0147555.

[15] Colvin, L., Leonard, S., Schiavello, T., Ellaway, C., Klerk, N., Christodoulou, J., Msall, M. and Leonard, S. (2003). Describing the phenotype in Rett syndrome using a population database. *Arch. Dis. Child,* 88 (1): 38 - 43. Accessed November 3, 2019. doi: 10.1136/adc.88.1.38.

[16] Julu, P. O., Engerstrom, I. W., Hansen, S., Apartopoulos, F., Engerstrom, B., Pini, G. et al. (2008). Cardiorespiratory challenges in Rett's syndrome. *Lancet,* 371 (9629): 1981 - 1983. Accessed November 3, 2019. doi: 10.1016/S0140-6736(08)60849-1.

[17] Young, D. J., Bebbington, A., Anderson, A., Ravine, D., Ellaway, C., Kulkami, A. et al. (2008). *The diagnosis of autism in a female: could it be Rett syndrome.* Accessed November 3, 2019. doi: 10.1007/s00431-007-0569-x.

[18] Ager, S., Fyfe, S., Christodoulou, J., Jacoby, P., Schmitt, L. And Leonard, H. (2006). Predictors of scoliosis in Rett syndrome. *J. Child*

Neurol., 21 (9): 809 - 813. Accessed November 3, 2019. doi: 10.1177/08830738060210091501.

[19] Lotan, M., Gootman, A. (2011). Regaining walking ability in individuals with Rett syndrome. *Int. J. Disabil. Hum. Dev.,* 11 (2): 163 - 169. Accessed November 3, 2019. doi: 10.1515/ijdhd-2012-0020.

[20] Larsson, G., Engerstrom, I. W. (2001). Gross motor ability in Rett syndrome-the power of expectation, motivation and planning. *Brain Dev.*, 23 (1): 77 - 81. Accessed November 3, 2019. doi: 10.1016/s0387-7604(01)00334-5.

[21] Lotan, M., Isakov, E. and Merrick, J. (2004). Improving functional skills and physical fitness in children with Rett syndrome. *J. Intellect. Disabil. Res.,* 48 (8): 730 - 735. Accessed November 3, 2019. doi: 10.1111/j.1365-2788.2003.00589.x.

[22] Budden, S. S., Gunness, M. E. (2003). Possible mechanisms of osteopenia in Rett syndrome: bone histomorphometric studies. *Journal of Child Neurology*, 18 (10): 698 - 702. Accessed November 3, 2019. doi: 10.1177/08830738030180100401.

[23] Velickovic, D. T., Perat, M. V. (2005). Basic principles of the neurodevelopmental treatment. *Medicina*, 42 (41): 112 - 120. Accessed November 3, 2019. http://www.bioline.org.br/pdf?me05016.

[24] Valvano, J., Rapport, M. (2006). Activity-focused motor interventions for infants and young children with neurological conditions. *Infants and Young children,* 19 (4): 292 - 307. Accessed November 3, 2019. doi:10.1097/00001163-200610000-00003.

In: Medical Care
Editor: Brian A. Soileau

ISBN: 978-1-53618-048-0
© 2020 Nova Science Publishers, Inc.

Chapter 3

THE INTERDISCIPLINARY APPROACH IN THE REHABILITATION OF PATIENTS WITH RETT SYNDROME

Alen Kapel[1], *Tine Kovacic*[1], *Tomaz Velnar*[1,2,*]
and Natasa Kos[1,3]

[1]Alma Mater Europaea-ECM Maribor, Maribor, Slovenia
[2]Department of Neurosurgery,
University Medical Centre Ljubljana, Ljubljana, Slovenia
[3]Department of Rehabilitational Medicine,
University Medical Centre Ljubljana, Slovenia

ABSTRACT

Rett syndrome is a rare genetic neurological syndrome, affecting almost only females and leading to severe impairments in all areas of the affected persons' life, including speech, mobility, posture, digestive and pulmonary function. Most distinct symptoms include stereotypical hand movements, ataxia and atrophy of lower limbs and signs of autism. The

---

[*] Corresponding Author's Email: tvelnar@hotmail.com.

neurological disorders in patients with Rett syndrome embrace various types of impairments or abnormalities, underlined by biochemical and structural abnormalities of brain, spinal cord and peripheral nerves. Clinically, these conditions may involve several disorders, including paralysis, spasticity, seizures, orthopaedic deformities, pain syndromes, disturbances of coordination, mobility and others. An interdisciplinary approach to neurological disorders demonstrated in Rett syndrome is therefore of utmost importance. The aim is to revert progressive deterioration with a wide spectrum and a combination of neurorehabilitational interventions. In order to examine the effects of complex interdisciplinary neurophysiotherapy, five girls with Rett syndrome were included in our experimental study. The GMFM-88 scale was used to determine the gross motor function prior and after habilitation. It was found that the interdisciplinary approach with combined neurophysiotherapy and continuous habilitation was very efficient in the gross motor function improvement in these patients, which has confirmed the importance of an interdisciplinary approach in the habilitation of the disease symptoms.

Keywords: Rett syndrome, interdisciplinary treatment, neurological rehabilitation, neurological disorder

INTRODUCTION

Rett syndrome (RS) is a rare genetic neurological syndrome that appears in young females due to the mutation of MECP2 gene and affects the grey matter of the brain [1]. It is known as a progressive neurodevelopmental disorder, involving molecular changes in the brain, which relate to neuropathological findings, although the scientifically proven neurochemical substate has yet to be defined [1, 2]. RS includes four stages of developmental regression with profound phenotypic features [3]. Stereotypical arm movement, regression of the gross motor function, microcephaly, epilepsy, regression with regards to the balance and protective reactions, spasticity, hypersensitivity, bradykinesia, dystonia, ataxia, apraxia tremor, cardiac dysfunction and postural irregularities are some of the most common phenotypic RS features [2-11]. At first, RS was considered an impairment in a form of autism, dementia, ataxia and loss of arm function [2-4].

Neurological and developmental disorders involve loss of speech and manual skills, inability to walk, apraxia, ataxia, epilepsy, respiratory insufficiency and disproportionate muscle tone, and inadequate visual perception of depth. A cognitive assessment in children with RS is difficult. However, children have a broad spectrum of moods and emotions [3, 9, 10]. The incidence of the syndrome is between 1:10.000 in new-born girls, regardless of race and other demographic features, apart from the gender [12].

In most cases, births of girls with RS happen without complications or other prenatal and perinatal distinctions [3]. Disproportions in muscle tone appear in the early developmental stage, which inhibit the ability to implement two-stroke climbing and consequently result in development of specific movement patterns. The typology of the MECP2 mutations plays a major role in the development of RS [9]. A large number of girls with RS live longer than 60 years, whereas the average life expectancy of girls with RS is a fraction lower compared to the healthy population. Incidence of sudden death is 25% higher than in healthy individuals [2]. The reason for this are disorders of the autonomic nervous system and cardiac instability. Parkinson's disease is also common at an older age [2, 3].

The purpose of this research was to study the effect of complex special neurophysiotherapeutic intervention on improving health conditions of girls with RS, in the area of gross motor function, defined and evaluated with the GMFM-88 scale. The main goal of the research was to study the minimal clinically important difference (MCID) in a 12-month neurophysiotherapeutic intervention aimed towards the improvement of gross motor function.

Rett Syndrome Mitigation

The aim of a neurological rehabilitation intervention is achieving relevant and important goals for an individual, with an active and dynamic educational process. In neurological rehabilitation, the focus of the process is on activities performed by disabled persons and goals striving towards independency [13]. Guidance, support and help are provided throughout the whole (re)habilitation process and are combined with different interventions carried out by medical and healthcare professionals [13, 14].

RS neurological status and neurological interventions are based on impairment, disability and handicap characteristics. Thus, impairment is the fundamental cause of a neurological investigation to recognise its dimensions and establish correct diagnosis. In neurological rehabilitation, professional intervention is not based only on impairment but on investigation of functional loss within the diagnosis. Functional implications of impairments are called disabilities, which impact the individual and try to be minimised during neurological rehabilitation [13, 14]. The aim of neurological rehabilitation is to reduce disability, gain skills with intent to maximise activity and to avoid or minimise implications as handicap [13].

An interdisciplinary approach is of utmost importance in neurological rehabilitation due to close involvement of different rehabilitation concepts, techniques and approaches [3, 13]. This also means that goals are not defined by a rehabilitation discipline but are based on needs and requirements of an individual in all aspects. Thus, the approaches and techniques are not only practised by neurophysiotherapists but must also be carried out by others who support the neurological rehabilitation team.

Neurophysiotherapists, occupational therapists, speech therapists, neurologists, physical therapists and paediatricians are almost always directly involved in inspection, evaluation, intervention and setting of re(habilitation) goals. Within neurophysiotherapy this means implementation of therapeutic concepts specifically intended for neurological illnesses. Intervention is based on preparation and guidance towards achieving normal development.

The direction of (re)habilitation interventions of children and adults with pathologies within the area of gross motor function is set in accordance with the medical and physiotherapeutic opinion, established by clinical paths and guidelines [3]. Inspections and interventions must be performed in a way that considers good foreign practice and most of all, the evaluation capacity and reaction monitoring of the observed individual. Due to the complexity of pathologies and the four regression phases, a thorough inspection with evaluation of achieved development milestones and complexity of neurological irregularities are required prior to intervention [3, 15]. the success and progress of intervention depends on the quality of performed inspection, which allows for an interdisciplinary habilitation approach aimed to maintain and improve functions of girls and to decrease the extent of pathologies [2, 3, 16].

Neurophysiotherapeutic intervention is necessary for girls with RS. Numerous traumas and deteriorations of condition are treated and prevented by specifically selected and applied therapies [3, 15, 16]. The main goals of intervention are to maintain and improve the motor function, develop and maintain the ability to transfer, decrease or prevent deformities, ease discomfort, decrease irritability and improve the level of independence [3, 17]. Therefore, an early discovery of pathological patterns is significant, since timely treatment allows quicker prevention of contractures and deformities, which would later at regression stage require orthopaedic procedures [18, 19]. Neurological situation sets the limit of intervention goals since learning correct movement patterns is only possible after normal righting musculature tone has been established [3, 17, 18]. Every girl with RS has her final intervention limits [3]. Intervention must be carried out rationally, without wasting time on intervention areas which are impossible to habilitate. The latter can only be achieved with professional interdisciplinary approach [3, 17, 19].

Intervention must be performed consistently, in an environment that stimulates movement and uses sensory and visual stimulations, until an achieved goal is established in a general motor pattern. [3, 18]. The extent of pathologies among girls varies. The differences can be found in both the physical characteristics and functions, as well as in actions and cooperation. Therefore, all interventions are personalised [14, 16-19].

Visual, vestibular and somatosensory systems maintain posture and balance, and along with musculoskeletal system provide gross motor function, therefore, the primary direction of intervention in case of RS is towards improvement of gross motor function [10]. The latter, based on cause and effect, improves cognitive function, skill, fine motor control and coordination. Physical activity has positive effects on concentration disorders [20].

Incorrect sensory and motor function development affects the entire development of a child, mainly sensory system, perceptive capability, cognitive status and psychological development. The latter causes an impaired perception of body and positions of extremities [3, 20].

DATA AND METHODS

In this research, the interdisciplinary approach with combined neurophysiotherapy and continuous habilitation in RS was studied. We have included 5 individuals diagnosed with RS for the period of 12 months.

Girls were selected randomly, according to the probability type sampling. All five girls come from one of the social institutions in Slovenia and have participated as part of intervention in seven specialists neurophysiotherapeutic treatments (Table 1). The relatively small sample size is the result of the low incidence of this syndrome in Slovenia. According to the data obtained by the neurological department of the paediatric clinic of the University Medical Centre Ljubljana, there are 18 girls diagnosed with RS in Slovenia, in 2020. In order to examine the effects of complex interdisciplinary neurophysiotherapy, five girls with RS were included in our experimental study. The GMFM-88 scale was used to determine the gross motor function prior, during and after habilitation. We used the gross motor function scale for assessment of gross motor function of people with RS (Gross Motor Function version 88 – GMFM-88).

Assessment scale: 0 = does not start, 1 = starts, 2 = partially performs, 3 = fully performs. 5 main chapters follow, which are divided into sub-chapters which will be used for assessment of patients. Scale limitations include:

- Scale is not suitable for individuals who show a high level of gross motor function since its range is limited,
- it assesses the extent and does not include the effect of environment on an individual and her daily activities,
- nor does it assess the quality of movement.

The study was carried out in accordance with the principles of International Code of Medical Ethics and the Helsinki/Tokyo Declaration. We have also obtained consensus of the Commission of the Republic of Slovenia for medical ethics (no. 0120-47/2018/4), and consensus of the Scientific Council of the Social and Security Institution which the patients are part of, as well as the consensus of their parents.

Table 1. Neurophysiotherapy treatment interventions

Reference number	1	2	3	4	5
Birth year	1993	1991	1991	1974	2001
Neurodevelopmental treatment	yes	yes	yes	yes	yes
Hippotherapy	no	yes	no	yes	yes
Physical therapy	no	no	yes	no	no
Active-assisted exercise program	yes	yes	yes	yes	yes
Endurance program	yes	yes	yes	yes	yes
Walking program	yes	yes	yes	yes	yes
Coordination exercise program	yes	yes	yes	yes	yes

Data was statistically processed using the SPSS software (Statistical Package for the Social Sciences 21). We have used the t-test. We used table and graphical demonstrations for presenting quantitative data.

RESULTS

In the study, five girls with diagnosed RS, aged between 18 and 45 (Mean = 29) participated in the gross motor function determination and neurophysiotherapy intervention. The GMFM-88 scale was used prior and after 12 months of habilitation which included seven specific personalised neurophysiotherapeutic interventions such as Bobath neurodevelopmental treatment, hippotherapy, physical therapy, active-assisted exercise program, endurance, walking and coordination exercise programs. The GMFM-88 scale is proven to be an effective and precise tool for assessment of motor function during habilitation. Considering its extensiveness, it can only be used by neurophysiotherapists with previous experience and does not provide results regarding the quality of movement and multidimensional movement characteristics. Their initial gross motor condition varied, thus all of the girls involved participated in at least five and in no more than seven specific personalised neurophysiotherapeutic interventions.

GMFM-88 evaluation (Table 2) consists of gross motor activities in five different dimensions. Regarding the dimensions, A, B and D, there are significant improvements in evaluation scores between the prior and subsequent habilitation intervention, although improvements are not statistically significant (A: $p = 0.072$; B: $p = 0.069$; D: $p = 0.061$). Although A, B and D do not show statistically significant improvements, these are obtained due to the difference in pre and post score values. On the other hand, the dimensions C and E showed significant improvements in score evaluation and scores were also statistically significant (C: $p = 0.021$; E: $p = 0.048$).

Due to the differences in scores and statistically significant results, the total score of GMFM-88 (Figure 1, Table 2) has significally improved in gross motor activities in all participating girls with RS. Improvements are also statistically significant due to the value p (p = 0.032). Therefore, it was found that the interdisciplinary approach with combined specific personalised neurophysiotherapy and continuous habilitation was very efficient in the gross motor function improvement in these patients.

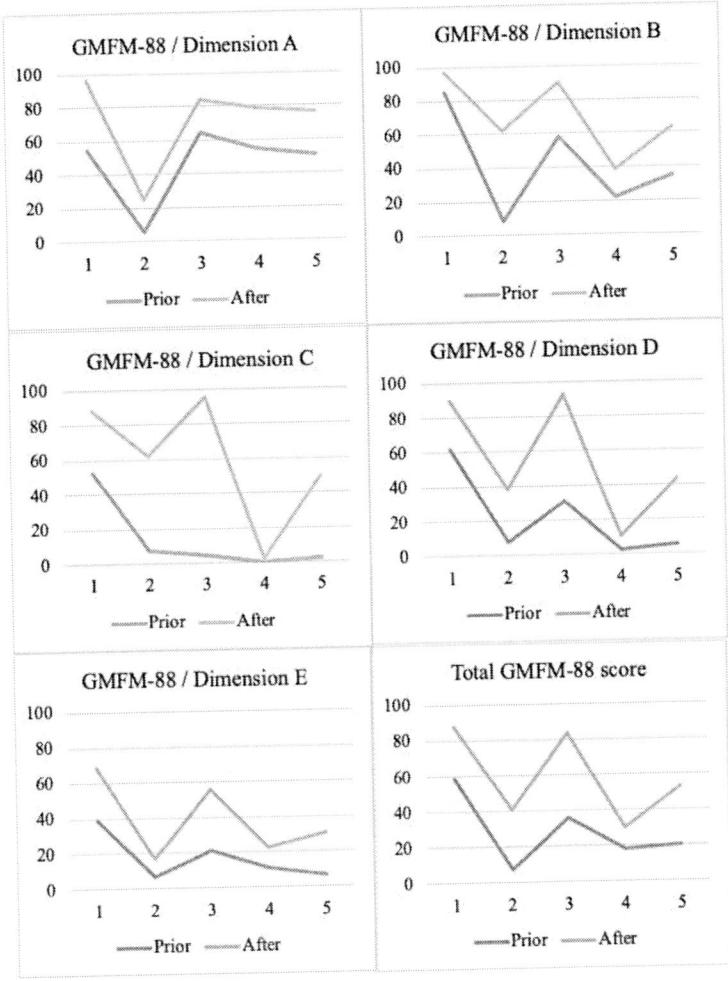

Figure 1. GMFM-88 evaluation.

Table 2. GMFM-88 evaluation in %

GMFM-88 dimension	Evaluation time	\multicolumn{5}{c}{Reference number of girl with RTT}				
		1	2	3	4	5
A	prior	54.90	5.88	64.70	54.90	50.98
	after	96.07	25.49	84.31	78.43	76.47
B	prior	85.00	8.33	58.33	21.67	35.00
	after	96.67	61.66	90.00	38.33	63.33
C	prior	52.38	7.14	4.76	0.00	2.38
	after	88.09	61.90	95.23	2.38	50.00
D	prior	61.50	7.69	30.77	2.56	5.12
	after	89.74	38.46	92.30	10.25	43.59
E	prior	38.88	6.94	20.83	11.11	6.94
	after	68.05	16.67	5.55	22.22	30.55
Total	prior	58.53	7.19	35.87	18.04	20.08
	after	87.72	40.83	83.47	30.32	52.78

DISCUSSION

RS involves a complex form of pathologies which due to their progressive-regressive combination and incidence of deformities, demands a broad spectrum of interventions. Inspection, evaluation and (re)habilitation procedures in particular segments demand an interdisciplinary, as well as multidisciplinary approach [21]. Neurophysiotherapeutic intervention is based on resolving irregularities in achieving realistic development goals, therefore, the purpose of intervention is to develop activity-related goals, activity-focused intervention and impairment-focused intervention [18, 22]. With this, we wish to preserve the existing gross muscle strength, maintain flexibility of upper and lower extremities, the existing ability to walk and improve the existing gross motor function [3, 13, 18, 22-25]. Due to the variability in reaching development stages, which the mutation type MECP2 depends on, the exact start of habilitation cannot be set. Thorough inspection and evaluation are significant, particularly the very familiar RS stages and criteria.

If possible, intervention must begin between the ages three and five (corrective age), because of the subsequent appearance of irregular motor patterns which become progressively dominant. Early implementation of rehabilitation allows for easier integration of proper motor function and decreases irregular motor patterns [3, 13, 18, 22-25]. An issue appears in case of already established irregular patterns or a prior increase of muscular tone, which additionally triggers the execution of irregular motor patterns in terms of gross motor function and posture which later results in appearance of deformities [13, 18, 22-24]. Brain lesions cause stereotypical motor patterns, which later effect extensory and synergy muscular groups [18, 26].

In our study, the intervention included seven different habilitation approaches for improving gross motor function (Table 1). Besides the common physiotherapeutic practice, we also implemented the neurodevelopmental evaluation (NE) as well as hippotherapy [18, 26]. NE inhibits pathological activity and triggers development of normal motor patterns since it optimizes individual's functions by improving control of body posture and selective movement. Hippotherapy is used for treating a wide range of diseases of neurological, orthopaedic or psychological origin, and has a positive effect on the gross motor function and function activity [10, 26]. GMFM-88 was used because it provides gross motor assessment for young individuals and individuals with severe motor disabilities. Studies conducted to date in the field of GMFM show multiple positive effects of the NE treatment, since they involve establishment of potential motor patterns in a form that a child is able to reach. Inhibition is used to decrease spasticity and to establish primary reflexes [27]. At first, the intervention involves inhibition of body and extremities' motor patterns, and later, the primary reflexes [27]. Facilitation techniques effect the improvement of head control, weight bearing of arms in balance reactions [27]. Habilitation procedure is focused on movement and righting reactions with the goal to inhibit worsening of bad posture and related expressed motor dysfunction, irregular head positioning and asymmetry of thoracic spine [23, 25, 27]. Asymmetric infant posture is formed through asymmetric motor patters, irregular shape of torso and unilateral head rotation [24]. Numerous studies analysing sitting have found that only one third of girls were able to independently sit on the floor or in a chair/wheelchair [6]. At the beginning, our sample showed that the sitting function was limited and that girls were unable to maintain their position due to underdeveloped or not developed righting techniques. There were improvements in both areas which were results of improved righting techniques and positioning of head and extremities when sitting. The study which focused on establishing improvements of gross motor function using NE, evaluated with the GMFM scale in children with CP discovered that, within 3 months, statistically significant differences were found in lying, sitting, crawling and kneeling, as well as in ability to stand [25].

The progress can also be further confirmed with studies from the field of hippotherapy which show that the use of hippotherapy in children with CP and other neurological typologies, positively effects the righting function and postural balance and consequently allows patients to achieve better condition with regards to gross motor function and functional activity [10, 28-30]. Most studies found that 10 to 12 treatments are required for improvement of postural characteristics, whilst some achieve significant progress after their first therapy, others only after 40 therapies [24]. There are also improvements in the area of strength and the range of motion which consequently shows in improved ability to walk and better static balancing [26]. Improved activation of flexors and torso extensors improves gross motor function of a child but the improvements are in most cases maintained for a period of three weeks, therefore, this is a lifetime habilitation [23]. In this case, they are using the therapeutic corset which limits appearance of contractures due to postural deterioration [25]. There were also improvements in lying and turning. Other studies also discovered similar findings [25, 31-34]. There were statistically significant differences with regards to turning, sitting and kneeling [31], a complete improvement of the gross motor function [32] and improvement of function movement [25].

Hippotherapy is a type of therapy that covers the fields of physiotherapy, occupation therapy and speech therapy and its goal is to use the movement of a horse to achieve sensory and motor integration. It is based on improving neurological functions and sensorimotor processes [35, 36]. According to an indication of presence of certain features of autism in girls, the research showed a wide spectrum of positive effects on characteristics of autism with regards to improvements in social integration and sensorimotor function and conduct [37, 38]. We have noticed that our sample experienced an improved environmental and habilitation awareness and a decreased sensory surplus. Tactile hypersensitivity of facial area is particularly addressed in studies showing the issue of hypersensitivity which corresponds with our findings [3]. Motor learning started to decrease the cognitive deficit which resulted in increased ability to focus and concentrate. Positive effects of physical activity on disruptions in concentration were also confirmed by other studies [3, 20]. Numerical frequency of impulse stereotypical arm movement was lower, the negative impact of external factors smaller, environment awareness improved, and the girls simultaneously became more perceptive of their environment and begun using intentional eye contact and grimaces, as well as laughter and occasional blinking.

When it comes to improving the gross motor function, the intervention does not only positively impact the muscular area but also other states, such as the vegetative and cognitive [22, 23, 31]. Diverse physical activity like walking and active exercises with passive stretching are part of the physiotherapeutic intervention [11]. Passive movement and active exercises allow a slower regression, improve cardiac function and contribute to preservation of bone density [11, 39]. Physical activity of girls with RS is also beneficial in case of issues with metabolism and cardiovascular status, mainly with regards to blood supply in lower extremities and a lower resting heart rate [40]. Studies have found that functional exercise has numerous positive effects on performance of daily activities which include the gross motor function [33].

General aspect of intervention presents progress particularly in the area of impulse stereotypical movements, left and right head rotation, improved sitting positions, improved righting technique and easier execution of manual action. Girls become more perceptive of environment, their uncontrolled impulsiveness decreases, improvements are found in concentration and coordinated movements and less frequent emotional outbursts. The latter has also been confirmed by studies, which pointed out that manual action can only be altered in a persistent environment enriched with motivation. The more independent girls are, the lesser the regression of manual action is [4].

This type of multidimensional interdisciplinary intervention is a prerequisite for progress in general, since its aimed at lowering the extent and intensity of pathologies in a complex manner and at improving vegetative function and subsequent habilitation participation.

Improvements of gross motor function are possible with a large number of treatments in short duration and neurophysiotherapists with specific skills [23]. Short duration and high frequency of therapies in children between 4 and 12 months of age, with posture and righting function irregularities, and motor dysfunctions [23]. Improvements in the area of gross motor function in girls affected by RS can be confirmed, since progress was made in all dimensions of habilitation. As far as the evaluation of the GMFM-88 goes, we can describe the state and the subsequent improvements in assessments of movements. However, the quality of execution cannot be evaluated. The latter presents the biggest issue in evaluation and reading of the evaluation reports based on GMFM-88. The scale would have to be amended and include certain criteria that would allow easier precise evaluation, such as the type of execution of movement and its quality, since numerous authors of similar studies pointed out the same issue with regards to data interpretation [25, 31-34]. Although the GMFM-88 scale allows measured evaluation of progress of gross motor function, behaviour monitoring is required for establishing multidimensional improvements.

The main issue of our study was the low level of RS incidence in Slovenia, therefore there were no statistically significant differences in certain chapters, despite the differences being identified in evaluation values.

Conclusion

The patients with RS improved their gross motor function, however, the functional status of improvements varies among the individuals. Some progressed faster than others. Habilitation of these girls is a lifetime procedure since just a one-week break from habilitation program can be detected. The individuals with RS in the existing study are considered persons with long-term, often progressive, decreased capability and disorders, therefore, a continuous habilitation is required, but not only in centralised rehabilitation institutions, but in special social security institutions for training, work and security for maintaining acquired motor skills and abilities and with it increased independence and autonomy. An interdisciplinary approach to neurological disorders demonstrated in RS is therefore of utmost importance.

References

[1] Kyle, M. S., Vashi, N. and Justice, M. J. (2018). Rett syndrome: a neurological disorder with metabolic components. *Open Biol,* 8 (2): 1-17. Accessed November 3, 2019. doi: 10.1098/rsob.170216.

[2] Percy, A. K. (2016). Progress in Rett syndrome: from discovery to clinical trials. *Wien Med Wochenschr,* 166 (11): 325-332. Accessed November 3, 2019. doi: 10.1007/s10354-016-0491-9.

[3] Lotan, M., Hanks, S. (2006). Physical therapy intervention for individuals with Rett syndrome. *The scientific world journal,* 187 (6): 1314-1338. Accessed November 3, 2019. doi: 10.1100/tsw.2006.187.

[4] Downs, J., Bebbington, A., Jacoby, P., Williams, A. M., Ghosh, S., Kaufmann, W. and Leonard, H. (2010). Level of purposeful hand function as a marker of clinical severity in Rett syndrome. *Dev Med Child Neurol,* 52 (9): 817-23. Accessed November 3, 2019. doi: 10.1111/j.1469-8749.2010.03636.x.

[5] Fehr, S., Downs, J., Bebbington, A. and Leonard, H. (2010). Atypical presentations and specific genotypes are associated with a delay in diagnosis in females with Rett syndrome. *Am J Med Genet A,* 0 (10): 2535-2542. Accessed November 3, 2019. doi: 10.1002/ajmg.a.33640.

[6] Borst, E. H., Townend, S. G., Eck, M., Smeets, E., Berg, M., Laan, A. and Curfs, G. L. (2018). Abnormal foot position and standing and walking ability in Rett syndrome. *J Dev Phys Disabil,* 30 (2): 281-295. Accessed November 3, 2019. doi: 10.1007/s10882-017-9585-6.

[7] Ager, S., Fyfe, S., Christodoulou, J., Jacoby, P., Schmitt, L. And Leonard, H. (2006). Predictors of scoliosis in Rett syndrome. *J Child Neurol,* 21 (9): 809-813. Accessed November 3, 2019. doi: 10.1177/08830738060210091501.

[8] Carter, P., Downs, J., Bebbington, A., Williams, S., Jacoby, P., Kaufmann, W. and Leonard, H.(2010). Stereotypical hand movements in 144 subjects with Rett syndrome from the population-based Australian database. *Movement disorders,* 25 (3): 282-288. Accessed November 3, 2019. doi: 10.1002/mds.22851.

[9] Fehr, S., Bebbington, A., Ellaway, C., Rowe, P., Leonard, H. and Downs, J. (2010). Altered attainment of developmental milestones influences the age of diagnosis of Rett syndrome. *J Child Neurology,* 0 (00): 1-8. Accessed November 3, 2019. doi: 10.1177/0883073811401396.

[10] Moraes, G. A., Copetti, F., Angelo, R., V. (2016) The effects of hippotherapy on postural balance and function ability in children with cerebral palsy. *J Phys Ther Sci,* 28 (1): 2220-2226. Accessed November 3, 2019. doi: 10.1589/jpts.28.2220.

[11] Du, Q., Zhou, X., Wang, X., Chen, Sun., Yang, X., Chen, N., Liang, J., Deng, W. and Sun, K. (2015). Passive movement and active exercise for very young infants with congenital heart diseases. *Du et*

al. *Trials,* 30 (16): 288. Accessed November 3, 2019. doi: 10.1186/s13063-015-0816-9.

[12] Weaving, L. S., Ellaway, C. J. and Christodoulou, J. G. (2005). Rett syndrome: clinical review and genetic update. *J Med Genet,* 42 (1): 1-7. Accessed November 3, 2019. doi: 10.1136/jmg.2004.027730.

[13] 18 new – Barnes, M. P. (2003). Principles of neurological rehabilitation. *J Neurol Neurosurg Psychiatry*, 74 (4): 3-7. Accessed November 3, 2019. doi: 10.1136/jnnp.74.suppl_4.iv3.

[14] Halbertsma, J., Heerkens, Y. F., Hirs, W. M., Vrankrijker, M. W., Dorine, V. R. C. D., Napel, H. T. (2000). International classification of impairments, disabilities and handicaps. *Disability & Rehabilitation,* 22 (3): 144-156. Accessed November 3, 2019. doi: 10.1080/096382800297006.

[15] Ellaway, C., Christodoulou, J. (2001). Rett syndrome: clinical characteristics and recent genetic advances. *Disabil Rehabil,* 23 (3-4): 98-106. Accessed November 3, 2019. doi: 10.1080/09638280 150504171.

[16] Cass, H., Reilly, S., Owen, L., Wisbeach, A., Weekes, L., Slonims, V., Wigram, T. and Charman, T. (2003). Findings from a multidisciplinary clinical case series of females with Rett syndrome. *Dev Med Child Neurol,* 45 (5): 325-337. Accessed November 3, 2019. doi: 10.1017/s0012162203000616.

[17] Larsson, G., Engerstrom, I. W. (2001). Gross motor ability in Rett syndrome-the power of expectation, motivation and planning. *Brain Dev,* 23 (1): 77-81. Accessed November 3, 2019. doi: 10.1016/s0387-7604(01)00334-5.

[18] Velickovic, D. T., Perat, M. V. (2005). Basic principles of the neurodevelopmental treatment. *Medicina,* 42 (41): 112-120. Accessed November 3, 2019. http://www.bioline.org.br/pdf?me05016.

[19] Colvin, L., Leonard, S., Schiavello, T., Ellaway, C., Klerk, N., Christodoulou, J., Msall, M. and Leonard, S. (2003). Describing the phenotype in Rett syndrome using a population database. *Arch Dis*

Child, 88 (1): 38-43. Accessed November 3, 2019. doi: 10.1136/adc. 88.1.38.

[20] Jacobsen, K., Viken, A. and Von Tetchner, S. (2001). Rett syndrome and aging: a case study. *Disabil Rehabil*, 23 (3-4): 160-166. Accessed November 3, 2019. doi: 10.1080/09638280150504234.

[21] Mount, R. H., Hastings, R. P., Reilly, S., Cass, H. and Charman, T. (2001). Behavioral and emotional features in Rett syndrome. *Disabil Rehabil*, 23 (3-4): 129-138. Accessed November 3, 2019. doi: 10.1080/09638280150504207.

[22] Lotan, M., Gootman, A. (2011). Regaining walking ability in individuals with Rett syndrome. *Int J Disabil Hum Dev,* 11 (2): 163-169. Accessed November 3, 2019. doi: 10.1515/ijdhd-2012-0020.

[23] Valvano, J., Rapport, M. (2006). Activity-focused motor interventions for infants and young children with neurological conditions. *Infants & Young children,* 19 (4): 292-307. Accessed November 3, 2019. doi:10.1097/00001163-200610000-00003.

[24] Arndt, W. S., Chandler, S. L., Mcelroy, J., Jane, K. S. and Sharkley, A. M. (2008). Effects of a neurodevelopmental treatment – based trunk protocol for infants with posture and movement dysfunction. *Pediatr Phys Ther,* 20 (1): 11-22. Accessed November 3, 2019. doi: 10.1097/PEP.0b013e31815e8595.

[25] Jung, W. M., Landenberger, M., Jung, T., Lindenthal, T. and Philippi, H. (2017). Vojta therapy and neurodevelopmental treatment in children with infantile postural asymmetry. *J Phys Ther*, 29 (2): 301-306. Accessed November 3, 2019. doi: 10.1589/jpts.29.301.

[26] Labaf, S., Shamsoddini, A., Hollisaz, M. T., Sobhani, V. and Shakibaee, A. (2015). Effects of neurodevelopmental therapy on gross motor function in children with Cerebral palsy. *Iran J Child Neurol,* 9 (1): 36-41. November 3, 2019. doi: PMC4515339.

[27] Koca, T. T., Ataseven, H. (2015). What is hippotherapy? The indications and effectiveness of hippotherapy. *North Clin Istanb*, 2 (3): 247-252. Accessed November 3, 2019. doi: 10.14744/nci.2016. 71601.

[28] Behzadi, F., Noroozi, H. and Mohamadi, M. (2014). The comparison of the neurodevelopmental-bobath approach with occupational therapy home program on gross motor function of children with Cerebral palsy. *JRSR*, 1 (1): 21-24. Accessed November 3, 2019. doi: 10.30476/JRSR.2014.41048.

[29] Shurtleff, T. L., Standeven, J. W. and Engsberg, J. R. (2009). Changes in dynamic trunk/head stability and functional reach after hippotherapy. *Arch Phys Med Rehabil,* 90 (7): 1185-1195. Accessed November 3, 2019. doi: 10.1016/j.apmr.2009.01.026.

[30] Casady, R. L. and Nichols, D. S. (2004). The effect of hippotherapy on ten children with cerebral palsy. *Pediatr Phys Ther*, 16 (3): 165-172. Accessed November 3, 2019. doi: 10.1097/01.PEP.0000136003. 15233.0C.

[31] Herrero, P., Asensio, A., Garcia, E. et al. (2010). Study of the therapeutic effects of an advanced hippotherapy simulator in children with cerebral palsy: a randomised controlled trial. *BMC Musculoskelet Disord*, 71 (11): 1-6. Accessed November 3, 2019. doi: 10.1186/1471-2474-11-71.

[32] Ketelaar, M., Vermeer, A., Hart, H., Petegem-van Beek, E., Helders, P. J. (2001). Effects of a functional therapy program on motor abilities of children with cerebral palsy. *Phys Ther*, 81 (9): 1534-1545. Accessed November 3, 2019. doi: 10.1093/ptj/81.9.1534.

[33] Shamsoddini, A. R. (2010) Comparison between the effect of neurodevelopmental treatment and sensory integration therapy on gross motor function in children with cerebral palsy. *Iran J Child Neurology*, 4 (1): 31-38. Accessed November 3, 2019. doi: https://doi.org/10.22037/ijcn.v4i1.1723.

[34] Akbari, A., Javad, M., Shahraki, S. and Jahanshahi, J. (2009). The effects of functional therapy on motor development in children with cerebral palsy. *Iran J Child Neurology*, 8 (4): 23-32. Accessed November 3, 2019. https://www.sid.ir/en/journal/ViewPaper.aspx?ID=169484.

[35] Arndt, S. W., Chandler, L. S., Sweeney, J. K., Sharkey, M. A. and McElroy, J. J. (2008). Effects of a neurodevelopmental treatment-

based trunk protocol for infants with posture and movement dysfunction. *Pediatr Phys Ther*, 20 (1):11-22. Accessed November 3, 2019. doi: 10.1097/PEP.0b013e31815e8595.

[36] Meregillano, G. (2004). Hippotherapy. *Phys Med Rehabil Clin N Am*, 15 (4): 843–854. Accessed November 3, 2019. doi: 10.1016/j.pmr.2004.02.002.

[37] Benda, W., McGibbon, N. H. and Grant, K. L. (2003). Improvements in muscle symmetry in children with cerebral palsy after equine-assisted therapy (hippotherapy). *J Altern Complement Med*, 9 (6): 817–825. Accessed November 3, 2019. doi: 10.1089/107555303771952163.

[38] Muslu, G. K. and Conk, H. (2011). Animal-assisted interventions and their practice in children. *Duehyo ED*, 4 (2): 83–88. Accessed November 3, 2019. https://scholar.google.com/scholar_lookup?journal=Duehyo+ED&title=Animal-Assisted+Interventions+and+Their+Practice+in+Children&author=GK+Muslu&author=H+Conk&volume=4&publication_year=2011&pages=83-8&.

[39] Ajzenman, H. F., Standeven, J. W. and Shurtleff, T. L. (2013). Effect of hippo- therapy on motor control, adaptive behaviors and participation in children with autism spectrum disorder: a pilot study. *Am J Occup Ther*, 67 (6): 653–663. Accessed November 3, 2019. doi: 10.5014/ajot.2013.008383.

[40] Lotan, M., Isakov, E., and Merrick, J. (2004). Improving functional skills and physical fitness in children with Rett syndrome. *J Intellect Disabil Res,* 48 (8): 730–735. Accessed November 3, 2019. doi: 10.1111/j.1365-2788.2003.00589.x.

[41] Lotan, M. and Zysman, L. (2006). The digestive system and nutritional considerations for individuals with Rett syndrome. *Scientific World Journal*, 6: 1737–1749. Accessed November 3, 2019. doi: 10.1100/tsw.2006.264.

In: Medical Care
Editor: Brian A. Soileau

ISBN: 978-1-53618-048-0
© 2020 Nova Science Publishers, Inc.

Chapter 4

THE ROLE OF ENDPLATE IN DEGENERATIVE DISC DISEASE TREATMENT: THE ISOLATION OF HUMAN CHONDROCYTES FROM VERTEBRAL ENDPLATE

Lidija Gradisnik[1,2], Uros Maver[1], Gorazd Bunc[3], Matjaz Vorsic[3], Janez Ravnik[3], Tomaz Smigoc[3], Roman Bosnjak[2,4] and Tomaz Velnar[2,3,4,*]

[1]Institute of Biomedical Sciences, Medical Faculty Maribor,
Maribor, Slovenia
[2]AMEU-ECM Maribor, Maribor, Slovenia
[3]Department of Neurosurgery, University Medical Centre Maribor,
Maribor, Slovenia
[4]Department of Neurosurgery, University Medical Centre Ljubljana,
Ljubljana, Slovenia

Abstract

Introduction. As a replacement option for laboratory animals, the *in vitro* organ culture systems are becoming increasingly essential. To study the possible mechanisms of intervertebral disc (IVD) degeneration, live disc cells are highly appealing. Especially the endplate plays an essential role in the degenerative disc disease. Although most intervertebral disc cells have been isolated from animal tissue, the experimental result cannot be conveyed from animals directly to humans. In order to study the degenerative processes of the endplate chondrocytes in vitro, we have established a relatively quick and easy protocol for isolation of human chondrocytes from the vertebral endplates.

Materials and Methods. The fragments of human lumbar endplate were obtained following lumbar fusion. The cartilaginous endplate fragments were collected, cut, grinded and partially digested with collagenase I. Sequential centrifugation and separation followed after enzymatic digestion, then the sediment was harvested and cells were seeded in suspension, supplemented with special media containing high nutrient level. Morphology was determined with phalloidin staining and the characterization for collagen I, collagen II and aggrecan with immunostaining.

Results. In appropriate laboratory conditions, the isolated cells retained viability and proliferated quickly. The confluent culture was obtained after 14 days. Six to 8 hours after seeding, attachments were observed and after 12 hours, proliferation of the isolated cells followed. The cartilaginous endplate chondrocytes were stable with the viability up to 95%.

Conclusion. Human chondrocyte cell culture allows the *in vitro* study of endplate cells. The reported cell isolation process is simple, economical and quick, allowing establishing a viable long-term cell culture. The availability of chondrocyte cell model will permit the study of cell properties, biochemical aspects, the potential of therapeutic candidates for the treatment of disc degeneration as well as toxicology studies in a well-controlled environment.

Keywords: intervertebral disc, endplate, degenerative disc disease, human chondrocytes, cell isolation

INTRODUCTION

Low back pain caused by the degenerative disease of the intervertebral disc is a chronic condition. It may result from numerous factors and represents one of the leading causes of disability and healthcare expenses in adults worldwide [1]. The disc generated pain and pain from chronic instability of the affected spine segments may in long term lead to significant functional disability in both genders, therefore considerably affecting living quality, especially in young and active population. The precise pathomorphological mechanism for the degenerative disease of the intervertebral disc still remains unknown. Several risk factors such as age, smoking, obesity and diabetes as well as several genetic, occupational and psychosocial factors have been identified. These known and unknown factors leading to disc degeneration are complex and frequently encompass synergistic interactions between biological and physical mechanisms [2-5].

The degenerative disc disease is a progressive and chronic disorder. On clinical imaging, the most important characteristics include visible changes in the nucleus pulposus, which is the first structure affected. The matrix degeneration and the intervertebral disc cell death occur first in the innermost part of the nucleus pulposus. The nucleus loses height and integrity, which may be seen on the magnetic resonance imaging (MRI) as alteration in the signal intensity. As a result of concomitant annular failure, the herniations of various degrees may occur. When speaking of intervertebral disc degeneration, the majority of investigation has been directed into the nucleus pulposus and annulus fibrosus, the most commonly affected structures of the intervertebral disc. The vertebral endplate role in these conditions, however, has frequently been overlooked. New studies have shown that this structure is at least equally important in the degenerative cascade as are the former two [6-9]. The purpose of this article is therefore to stress the importance of the vertebral endplate function in the intervertebral disc health and disease and to describe an improved protocol for the endplate chondrocyte isolation for the purpose of the *in vitro* disc degeneration research.

THE ANATOMY OF VERTEBRAL ENDPLATE

The intervertebral disc is an avascular fibrocartilaginous structure, which is located between two neighbouring vertebrae. It provides load transmission and flexibility throughout the spinal column [10]. It is composed of three distinct layers: I) the central nucleus pulpous with its outer and inner part, II) the collagenous annulus fibrous, circumferentially surrounding the nucleus and III) the cartilaginous terminal plates or endplates, separating the annulus fibrosus and nucleus pulposus form the vertebral bodies [10-12].

The endplates are composed of two parts, the outer bony endplate and the inner cartilaginous endplate [12]. The bony endplate passes into the vertebral bone on one side and into the cartilaginous plate on the other, which borders to the intervertebral disc, namely the annulus and the nucleus. The structural function of the cartilaginous part is the separation of the intervertebral disc from the adjacent vertebrae and to contain the nucleus pulposus. The cartilage endplate is composed of semi-porous thickened cancellous bone of 0.6 mm to 1 mm in thickness that is arranged in layers and of hyaline cartilage of 0.2 mm to 0.8 mm in thickness. The thickness of the human endplate diminishes toward the centre. The extracellular substance of the cartilaginous endplate, which is the most abundant component, consists mainly of water proteoglycans, the main constituent being aggrecan, and type II collagen. The collagen fibres of the cartilaginous part of the endplate are mostly aligned parallel to the vertebral surface, in contrast to the erratic pattern of collagen alignment found in the articular cartilage. The water content varies during the lifetime; it is close to 80% after birth and then diminishes to below 70% after 15 years of age [13-15].

Where the endplate integrates with the annulus, it has a more complex structure. In the region of the outer annulus, the vertebral boundary is formed by a fibrocartilaginous bondage where the annular fibres are inserted into an area of calcified cartilage that is anchored to the subchondral bone [9, 12]. The collagen fibres located in the lamellae of the inner part of the annulus fibrosus run in continuity with the collagen fibres in the endplate, thus minimising the stress concentrations during complex loading that includes compression, tension and shear forces. The cartilaginous part of the endplate is structurally not fixed into the bony part and therefore this interface may be separated easily [16-18].

The cartilage endplate encompasses the inferior and superior boundaries of the intervertebral disc and forms its main nutrient supply network. The bony endplate runs into the bone marrow compartment of the vertebra, which contains thin-walled capillaries, haematopoietic cells, fat cells and nerves [19, 20]. The vertebral capillaries and nerves that enter the basivertebral foramen at the posterior vertebral cortex supply this area through the small pores located in the cortical shell. In the centre, the capillaries form an arterial network, which then branches and terminates nearby the cartilaginous endplate. These vessels and sinusoid venous channels make a continuous vascular bed across the bone-disc interface. This enables the disc nutrition by diffusion from the vessels in the vicinity. As decreased nutrient supply is one of the factors that are associated with the degenerative process of the intervertebral disc, it is understandable that the changes in the cartilage endplate also display a noticeable effect on the disc degeneration [11, 17].

The nerve supply of the vertebral endplate is comparable to that of the intervertebral disc *per se*. The nerve endings are located mainly in the outer layers of the endplate and spread to its central part. In a healthy disc, they extend approximately to the three outermost lamellae of the annulus fibrosus. Ninety percent of the nerves consist of sympathetic afferent fibres and are branches of the sinuvertebral nerves. In pathological conditions, their concentration is increased in the areas of endplate damage. These nerves can send nociceptive impulses to the sympathetic nervous system that may cause a form of visceral-like pain, which may be similar to the enteric structures [13, 18, 21, 22].

The Degenerative Process of the Vertebral Endplate

Intervertebral disc degeneration is many times related to low back pain [12, 17]. The surrounding tissues of the intervertebral disc are normally included in mechanical and biochemical homeostasis, which are disturbed during the degenerative events. Besides the intervertebral disc itself, included are also the cartilaginous endplate, bony vertebral endplate and the adjacent vertebral bodies, which are in contact through the endplates [18]. The transmission of mechanical loads on the intervertebral disc is largely influenced by vertebral bodies and bone in the vertebral endplate. This load transmission therefore depends on both the morphological properties of the bone and its composition. The former includes the properties and strength of the cortical and trabecular bone and the latter the bone mineral density. As a result, the preservation of disc health is dependent on the structure and composition of these surrounding tissues, since the changes in surrounding tissues may induce cellular, molecular and structural disorders in the intervertebral disc [22-24]. With aging, the disc extracellular matrix and disc cells undergo significant biologic changes that are involved in the process of the intervertebral disc degeneration. The main factor is the loss of proteoglycans. These large molecules are being degraded to smaller fragments that are lost from the disc tissue. The consequence is the fall in the osmotic pressure in the disc matrix and subsequent loss of water molecules. All these events affects mechanical properties of the disc, eventually causing disc bulging and height loss [25, 26].

The degenerative processes of the intervertebral disc, endplate and adjacent bone marrow are highly associated [25]. It is well known that the degenerative disc disease has been strongly associated to the endplate alterations of bone composition and morphology, however, the exact aetiology and causative relationship between the progression of degenerative disc disease and endplate changes have not yet been fully understood. Various alterations in endplate morphology due to degenerative disc disease have been observed. Some researchers reported increased porosity of the endplate, thinning of its layers and loss of the tissue strength, while others have observed that with the increasing severity of disc degeneration, the vertebral bone mineral density increased and resulted in the calcification and thickening of the endplate during the progression of the disc degeneration [27, 28]. During the progression of intervertebral disc disease, the breakdown of the extracellular matrix in the cartilage endplate is among the most important processes. The degenerative processes affecting the disc encompasses also other structures in the vicinity, ultimately influencing the vertebral endplate and the vertebral bone, since the endplate and bone marrow are highly associated [27-30].

Similarly to the macromolecules breakdown in the nucleus pulposus, the degradation of aggrecan and collagen II are viewed as a central feature in the damage of the cartilage endplate during the course of degeneration. Here, the matrix metalloproteinases are principal enzymes for collagen breakdown [31]. The degenerated cartilage endplate is also a source of inflammatory mediators, including interleukin-1β, tumour necrosis factor (TNF)-α, macrophage inhibition factor and interleukin-6. The proteoglycan loss affects movement of other molecules into and out of the extracellular matrix as well. Serum proteins and cytokines diffuse into the matrix, affecting the cells and accelerating the process of the degeneration. The changes in the bone of the vertebral body have also been observed, in addition to the endplate morphology alterations. The variations in vertebral trabecular architecture depend on the severity of the disc degeneration. The intervertebral disc is therefore not the only and the most important structure in the spinal degenerative process. According to this data, the critical role of the vertebral endplate in the intervertebral disc health and degeneration is becoming increasingly apparent [32-36].

TREATMENT OF THE DEGENERATIVE DISC DISEASE

Beside conservative treatment, the most common currently available treatment for the degenerative disc disease remains operative [37-39]. This includes various procedures such as discectomy, spinal fusion, disc arthroplasty and epidural steroid injections. These options are in general considered interventional and none has been shown to reverse the degeneration cascade. The suppression of accelerated senescence and excessive apoptosis of disc cells may be another option to tackle the disc degeneration. Among current biologic therapies, gene-based therapy has been tried, as well as the use of mesenchymal stem cells, anti-catabolic factors, biomaterials and intradiscal infiltration of plasma rich in growth factors. When taking into account the biologic therapy in order to repair or regenerate the degenerated disc, nutrient and biomechanical factors should always be kept in mind, since they are the major causes of the biologic changes in the disc environment. The majority of these approaches still remain experimental and are not currently approved for everyday clinical use practice [40-45].

THE ISOLATION OF HUMAN CHONDROCYTES FROM VERTEBRAL ENDPLATE

As a replacement option for laboratory animals, the *in vitro* organ culture systems are becoming increasingly interesting [46, 47]. The techniques of *in vitro* cell cultures have made great advances in the recent years. Various cell models that involve isolated cells allow the study of physiological and pathophysiological mechanisms with no need for laboratory animals. Human cell cultures are indeed more suitable for the experiments concerning the human pathobiology and live cells in the *in vitro* organ systems are therefore becoming more and more appealing. Although most intervertebral disc cells have been isolated from animal tissue, the experimental result cannot be conveyed from animals directly to humans. In order to study the degenerative processes of the endplate chondrocytes *in vitro*, we have established a suitable protocol for isolation of human chondrocytes from the vertebral endplates [44, 48].

The endplate plays an essential role in the process of the intervertebral disc degeneration [28]. The chondrocytes in the endplates are the cells that are prone to degeneration during the intervertebral disc wear and tear, among other cells that constitute the disc, as are annulus fibrosus and nucleus pulposus cells. This is the reason that considering the endplate degeneration in the setting of the degenerative disc disease is becoming increasingly important. In the *in vitro* setting, numerous mechanical and biological aspects in a well-controlled physiological and mechanical environment can be studied on these cells. Human endplate chondrocytes can be obtained in higher numbers relatively easily from vertebral endplate that has been removed during various lumbar or cervical operations, addressing the degenerative spinal and intervertebral disc pathology [42, 49, 50]. Our group has established a relatively quick and easy protocol for vertebral endplate chondrocyte isolation with a high yield of cells and a low risk for contamination.

MATERIALS AND METHODS

The Source of Tissue

Tissue samples for cartilaginous endplate chondrocyte isolation was acquired during operations on lumbar spine. When lumbar stabilisation was needed, the intervertebral disc was removed and the cartilaginous endplates were thinned until the cortical bone of the vertebra was visible. In sterile conditions, the larger fragments of cartilaginous layer measuring about 1 cm^2 were transferred into the saline and transferred to the laboratory. The permission for human tissue utilisation has been obtained from the ethical committee as well as written informed consent form the patient.

Reagents

All materials and chemicals utilised in the experiments were of a laboratory grade. Advanced DMEM/F12 and other materials for cell culture were acquired from Thermo Fisher Scientific (Waltham, Massachussets, USA). Heat inactivated foetal bovine serum was purchased from Gibco (by Thermo Fisher Scientific, Waltham, Massachussets, USA). Streptomycin, penicillin, L-glutamine, phosphate-buffered saline (PBS), bovine serum albumin (BSA), Tween 20 and trypsin-EDTA were bought from Sigma-Aldrich (Merck KGaA, Darmstadt, Germany). Anti-Aggrecan antibody, Anti-Collagen 1 antibody, Anti-Collagen 2 antibody, Rabbit Anti-Mouse IgG H&L secondary antibody Alexa Fluor 488, Goat anti-rabbit IgG (H+L) secondary antibody Alexa Fluor 594, CytoPainter Phalloidin-iFluor 555 Reagent and Fluoroshield Mounting Medium With DAPI were from AbCam (Cambridge, UK) and Fixation solution (5x) from Millipore (Merck, Millipore, Darmstadt, Germany). All other substances were acquired from standard commercial suppliers.

The Preparation of Tissue for Cell Culture

In the cell laboratory, the fragments of viable tissue were transferred from transport centrifuge tubes into the petri dishes of 3.5 cm in diameter and washed with PBS. The collected tissue fragments weighted 0,324 g. The tissue was cut into smaller fragments of approximately 1 mm^3 with a No. 11 scalpel and incubated with collagenase 1 (2 mg/ml collagenase 1 in Advanced DMEM/F12 with 5% FBS) for 19 hours in controlled atmosphere (at 37° C and in 5% CO_2). As the tissue fragments were not digested completely, the suspension was filtrated through a 70 μm pore size mesh and centrifuged for 5 minutes at 400 x g. The sediment was then resuspended in 20 ml of Advanced DMEM with 100 IU/ml penicillin, 0.1 mg/ml streptomycin, 2 mM L-glutamine and 5% FBS and transferred into two T25 flasks. The growth medium was changed every three days.

Cell Characterisation

After the cell culture was obtained, chondrocytes from the cartilaginous endplate were characterised for the presence of aggrecan, collagen 1 and collagen 2. The cell morphology was appreciated with the actin cytoskeleton staining. After characterisation, the Mounting medium with DAPI was utilised for nuclei staining.

Into the wells of P24 plates, round cover glasses of 12 mm in diameter were placed. The first passage cell suspension with 50000 cells per well was added. The incubation in controlled atmosphere at 37° C and in 5% CO followed; two days for actin cytoskeleton staining and 13 days for aggrecan, collagen 1 and collagen 2 staining. In both cases, the medium was discarded and cell monolayer quickly washed with PBS. The cells were then fixed with the Fixation solution (1:5 in Milliq water) for 15 minutes at room temperature. Triple irrigation with cold PBS followed.

A) For staining of the actin cytoskeleton, the standard manufacturer's protocol was followed. Briefly, the fixed cells were washed with cold PBS and after the last washing, the working solution of conjugated phalloidin was added (1:1000 in PBS with 1% BSA). The cells were incubated for 90 minutes at room temperature and then washed with the PBS three times for 5 minutes. Then, the cells were washed again with the Milliq water and two drops of Mounting Medium with DAPI were added. Images were taken at x10 magnification on EVOS FL fluorescence microscope (Thermo Fisher Scientific, Waltham, Massachussets, USA) (Ex/Em = 556/574 nm).

B) For aggrecan, collagen 1 and collagen 2 staining, the cells were incubated after the last PBS irrigation for 30 minutes with the PBS solution (PBS with 1% BSA and 0.1% Tween 20 for blockade of nonspecific antibodies). Primary antibodies in solution containing PBS with 1% BSA and 0.1% Tween 20 were added; I) for aggrecan, the Anti-Aggrecan antibody (1:50), II) for collagen 1, the Anti-Collagen 1 antibody (1:500) and III) for collagen 2, the Anti-Collagen 2 antibody (1:200). The cells were incubated overnight at 4° C. After triple irrigation with PBS for five minutes, the cells were incubated in the dark at room temperature for one hour with secondary antibodies. The following dilutions in PBS with 1%

BSA of secondary antibodies were used: for aggrecan 1:1000 Rabbit Anti-Mouse IgG H&L (Alexa Fluor 488) preadsorbed and for both collagens 1:1000 Goat Anti-Rabbit IgG H&L (Alexa Fluor 594). Finally, the cells were washed three times for five minutes with PBS and after the last irrigation with Milliq water, two drops of Fluoroshield Mounting Mediuma with DAPI were added. Images were taken at x10 magnification on EVOS FL fluorescence microscope (Thermo Fisher Scientific, Waltham, Massachussets, USA) (for ggrecan Ex/Em = 495/519, for both collagens Ex/Em = 590/617).

RESULTS

The cell culture of cartilaginous endplate described in the experiment consisted of rapidly growing cells that were isolated from lumbar spine of an adult donor. The primary cell culture was 100% confluent after 14 days. From one T25 cell flask, approximately 1800000 cells were obtained. These were then split in ratio 1:3 and after six days, a 100% confluent culture of the first passage was obtained. These cells were named the CEP-1 (Cartilaginous Endplate Chondrocytes 1) (Figure 1). A part of these cells was stored in liquid nitrogen. A viability of more than 95% was observed when the cells were thawed and reseeded. The first passage cells were also used for characterisation, as described above.

The examination of the morphological properties after phalloidin staining showed a distinctive appearance of the isolated CEP-1. The characteristic nucleus shape was round with cells adopting round to triangular as well as elongated shape, which of course varied during the isolating process, depending on the attachment and growth phases. After a few days, the cells attached to the substrate and shape alterations were visible during this time. During the experiment, the cells were easy to maintain in the culture and were growing well. When a confluent culture was reached, the growth stopped due to the contact inhibition.

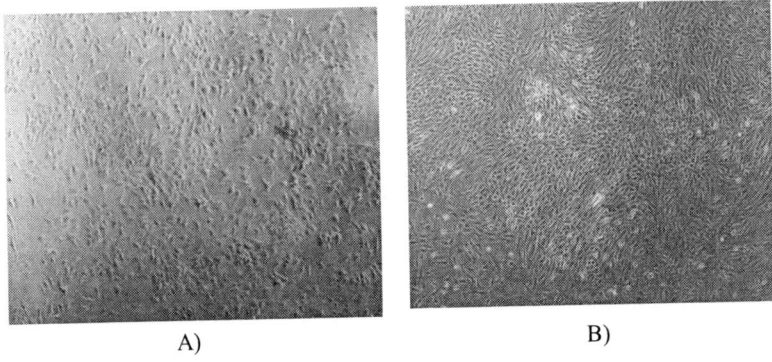

Figure 1. The primary culture of cartilaginous endplate cells. A) Eight days after the isolation, a low-density culture with individual round to polygonally shaped cells was evident. B) Two weeks after the isolation, the cells completely cover the flask surface with the formation of strong intercellular connections. Images were taken at x50 magnification on Zeiss Axiovert 40 inverted microscope. Scale bar = 200 µm.

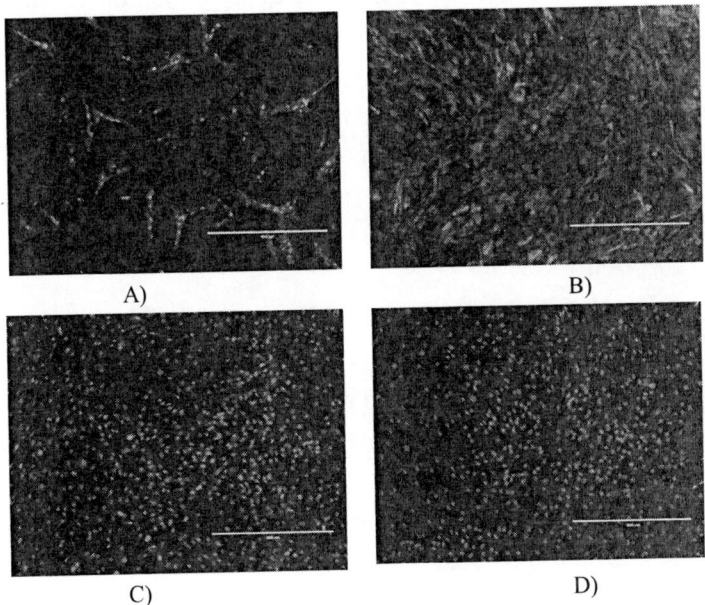

Figure 2. The immunocytochemical characterization of cartilaginous endplate cells in the first passage. A) The cell morphology was characterised using an orange fluorescent phalloidin conjugate that selectively binds to actin filaments (red). In low-density cultures, the cells show round to polygonal shape with actin filaments in the cytoplasm. B) The cells positive for aggrecan are green. C) The presence of collagen 2 and D) collagen 1 are demonstrated in red colour. Nuclei were counter-stained with DAPI (blue). Images were taken at x10 magnification on EVOS FL fluorescence microscope. Scale bar = 400 µm.

As aggrecan and collagens represent the main components of endplate chondrocytes, we have characterised the CEP-1 cells for these markers. The immunocytochemical staining methods were employed. It was confirmed that more than 90% of cultured cells from the first passage expressed the hondrocytic markers such as aggrecan, collagen 2 and collagen 1. This presence of the tested proteins therefore confirmed that the isolated culture consisted of the CEP-1 cells (Figure 2).

DISCUSSION

The vertebral endplate is one of the key elements of the disc stricture and the endplate chondrocytes are one of the key cells involved in the disc degeneration process [12, 16]. They have many important functions under physiological and pathological circumstances, including the metabolic support, role in the homeostasis of the extracellular environment, the maintenance of the extracellular matrix and nutrition of the discal nucleus and annulus beneath. It is therefore not surprising that the endplate cells have been of significant interest from multiple perspectives, including growth, development, degeneration, remodelling, repair and treatment strategies [15, 20].

As the intervertebral disc is the biggest avascular organ, the nutrition of the cells in the nucleus depend only on diffusion through the capillary network and spouts from the adjacent vertebral body [20, 22]. The cartilaginous endplate is also involved in the angiogenesis and damage to the one-cartilage surface may lead to altered matrix metabolism, which as a result has detrimental effects on the intervertebral disc. Having such important roles, the endplate chondrocytes represent an important target for basic and translational neuroscience research, especially for the *in vitro* cell models, concerned with the intervertebral disc degeneration [45]. Preserving the structural intcgrity and the function of the adjacent structures, including the vertebrae and endplates, may therefore protect the disc against degeneration.

The primary cell cultures of vertebral endplate chondrocytes have been isolated from various animal sources. In spite of a rich experimental portfolio, considerable differences between animal and human endplate chondrocytes exist [51-53]. Many other sources of vertebral tissue exist, every with its advantages and drawbacks. Human cells have the benefit of more accurately capturing the intervertebral disc environment. Therefore, these cells are widely used for the studies of spine physiology and metabolic processes in the intervertebral disc that would otherwise not be possible *in vivo*. Because many translational research projects aim to identify mechanisms that eventually lead to diagnostic and therapeutic approaches to target human diseases, chondrocytes are needed that better reflect the human intervertebral disc [54]. The animal cell models cannot be translated directly to humans and these differences are the main factor for further developing and improving the isolation methods and promoting the studies on human vertebral endplate chondrocytes. Therefore, endplate chondrocyte cultures obtained from human may respond more reliably and may help to elucidate the role of these cells in *in vivo* situations [28, 55].

There are not many reports about human vertebral endplate chondrocytes isolation. The isolation process is demanding, the cultures of these cells are poorly studied and could thus represent an important tool for understanding their functions [56, 57]. Therefore, we have developed a highly enriched primary endplate chondrocyte culture from adult specimen, obtained during neurosurgical spinal operations of the degenerative spine pathology. We have decided for the resection specimen of the cartilaginous endplates due to tissue accessibility in patents, treated for various degenerative spinal pathology. Especially suitable were the operations, where vertebral endplate needs to be removed or thinned, as is the case in the lumbar fusion. Here, large fragments of the cartilaginous endplate can be dissected when the intervertebral disc space is cleared and the endplate layers smoothened before the intervertebral implant preparation. In such cases, large cartilaginous areas represent an ideal source for the cell isolation, as they contain a large number of cells and the isolation process is therefore more successful. Simple discectomies (microfenestrations) are not so suitable for the samples, since here, the nucleus pulposus of the intervertebral disc is only emptied and no access to the endplates is gained. Additionally, the cervical endplate fragments taken during the anterolateral approach for cervical desis are also appropriate [57]. In both sources, namely lumbar and cervical, the cell density, cell population and dimensions are similar. Since the aim was to isolate untransformed cultures of human vertebral endplate chondrocytes, it was necessary to obtain a suitable part of the intervertebral disc, thus making it a perfect sample for the isolation process.

In the course of the cell isolation, it was necessary to develop an effective technique for the maintenance of cell culture, which is often challenging and complicated, so it may take long to establish an efficient and reliable culture, allowing the cells to maintain the characteristics of the tissue they originated from [45, 54, 55]. Despite the ideal characteristics, in contrast to transformed cell lines, the untransformed cell culture can dedifferentiate and the cells lose their phenotypic characteristics after a certain number of passages, depending on the cell type. This can be somewhat corrected by special conditions of cultivation and selective cell media [56].

The cartilaginous endplate cells exhibit a rounded morphology that is similar to that of articular chondrocytes. However, both differ substantially according to their cell markers [15]. Our endplate chondrocytes have retained the characteristics of the tissue, which they were isolated from. When observed under the light microscope during growth, the cells were pale-staining, exhibiting oval to round nuclei with little discernible cytoplasm. The cells were cultivated in flasks in a single layer. After the formation of confluent culture, the growth stopped. Cells did not accumulate in domes or grew in several layers. This indicates that the contact inhibition was maintained, which is unique for the untransformed cells and is not seen in cancer lines [58, 59]. The proliferation index of our isolated cells was high, which enabled a rapid formation of confluent cell culture.

The phenotypical characterisation of the cultured cells was performed with immunocytochemistry for the presence of key cell markers. The identification of specific markers defining various cell types in the intervertebral disc is important in order to characterise these cells and to define their phenotype. Unlike the markers of nucleus pulposus and annulus fibrosus cells, which have been defined, the cartilaginous endplate chondrocytes have no exactly recognised cell markers [15, 60, 61]. According to some reports, the markers, which are the cell products of the matrix component on the endplate, may change over the cell growth period, including the maturation and senescence of the endplate cells. Aggrecan and collagen have been described as the main components of both the cartilaginous endplate chondrocytes and other tissues, but their synthetic profiles are very different [62]. This means that the amount of the proteins verse during the cell life cycle. Immunocytochemistry on our isolates has confirmed the presence of collagen 1, collagen 2 and aggrecan, which is consistent also with the literature reports [15, 62].

We have established the isolation process to develop a highly enriched endplate chondrocyte culture from the adult endplate cartilage. The examination of morphological properties illustrated that the CEP-1 demonstrated typical chondrocyte appearance and cellular division to confluence. The described protocol for endplate chondrocytes isolation offers the opportunity to characterise these cells' functions *in vitro* and provides a valuable tool for studying the intervertebral disc degeneration process.

CONCLUSION

The demonstrated isolation process is simple, quick and economical, allowing to establish a long-term primary endplate chondrocyte cell culture. Cultured cells expressed characteristic markers and may represent an important new tool for the *in vitro* and *in vivo* studies. The availability of such system will permit the study of cell properties, biochemical aspects and the potential of therapeutic candidates for treatment of the intervertebral disc degeneration in a well-controlled environment on a human cell culture.

REFERENCES

[1] Lemeunier, N., Leboeuf-Yde, C., Gagey, O. (2012). The natural course of low back pain: a systematic critical literature review. *Chiropr Man Therap*, 20: 33.

[2] Hestbaek, L., Leboeuf-Yde, C., Manniche, C. (2003). Low back pain: what is the long-term course? A review of studies of general patient populations. *Eur Spine J*, 12: 149-165.

[3] Junge, T., Wedderkopp, N., Boyle, E., Kjaer, P. (2019). The natural course of low back pain from childhood to young adulthood - a systematic review. *Chiropr Man Therap*, 27: 10.

[4] Niënhaus, B. E. C., van de Laar, F. A. (2017). Lower back pain: understanding it is more important than treating it. *Ned Tijdschr Geneeskd*, 161: 2032.

[5] Morlion, B. (2013). Chronic low back pain: pharmacological, interventional and surgical strategies. *Nat Rev Neurol*, 9: 462-473.

[6] Kos, N., Gradisnik, L., Velnar, T. (2019). A brief review of the degenerative intervertebral disc disease. *Med Arch*, 73: 421-424.

[7] Iatridis, J. C., Nicoll, S. B., Michalek, A. J., Walter, B. A., Gupta, M. S. (2013). Role of biomechanics in intervertebral disc degeneration and regenerative therapies: what needs repairing in the disc and what are promising biomaterials for its repair? *Spine J*, 13: 243-262.

[8] Molladavoodi, S., McMorran, J., Gregory, D. (2020). Mechanobiology of annulus fibrosus and nucleus pulposus cells in intervertebral discs. *Cell Tissue Res*, 379: 429-444.

[9] Liu, C., Yang, M., Liu, L., Zhang, Y., Zhu, Q., Huang, C., et al. (2020). Molecular basis of degenerative spinal disorders from a proteomic perspective. *Mol Med Rep*, 21: 9-19.

[10] Chen, L., Battié, M. C., Yuan, Y., Yang, G., Chen, Z., Wang, Y. (2020). Lumbar vertebral endplate defects on magnetic resonance images: prevalence, distribution patterns, and associations with back pain. *Spine J*, 20: 352-360.

[11] Amelot, A., Mazel. C. (2018). The intervertebral disc: Physiology and pathology of a brittle joint. *World Neurosurg*, 120: 265-273.

[12] Tomaszewski, K. A., Saganiak, K., Gładysz, T., Walocha, J. A. (2015). The biology behind the human intervertebral disc and its endplates. *Folia Morphol (Warsz)*, 74: 157-168.

[13] Cheung, K. M., Orlansky, A. S., Sen, K., Elliot, D. M. (2009). Reduced nucleus pulposus glycosaminoglycan content alters intervertebral disc dynamic viscoelastic mechanics. *J Biomech*, 42: 1941-1946.

[14] Colombini, A., Lombardi, G., Corsi, M. M., Banfi, G. (2008). Pathophysiology of the human intervertebral disc. *Int J Biochem Cell Biol*, 40: 837-842.

[15] Pattappa, G., Li, Z., Peroglio, M., Wismer, N., Alini, M., Grad, S. (2012). Diversity of intervertebral disc cells: phenotype and function. *J Anat*, 221: 480-496.

[16] Sharifi, S., Bulstra, S. K., Grijpma, D. W., Kuijer, R. (2015). Treatment of the degenerated intervertebral disc; closure, repair and regeneration of the annulus fibrosus. *J Tissue Eng Regen Med*, 9: 1120-1132.

[17] Chan, W. C., Sze, K. L., Samartzis. D, Leung, V. Y., Chan, D. (2011). Structure and biology of the intervertebral disk in health and disease. *Orthop Clin North Am*, 42: 447-464.

[18] Jaumard, N. V., Welch, W. C., Winkelstein, B. A. (2011). Spinal facet joint biomechanics and mechanotransduction in normal, injury and degenerative conditions. *J Biomech Eng*, 133: 71010.

[19] Chen, C., Zhou, T., Sun, X., Han, C., Zhang, K., Zhao, C., et al. (2020). Autologous fibroblasts induce fibrosis of the nucleus pulposus to maintain the stability of degenerative intervertebral discs. *Bone Res*, 8: 7.

[20] Pattappa, G., Li, Z., Peroglio, M., Wismer, N., Alini, M., Grad, S. (2012). Diversity of intervertebral disc cells: phenotype and function. *J Anat*, 221: 480-496.

[21] Lundon, K., Bolton, K. (2001). Structure and function of the lumbar intervertebral disk in health, aging, and pathologic conditions. *J Orthop Sports Phys Ther*, 31: 291-306.

[22] Urban, J. P., Smith, S., Fairbank, J. C. (2004). Nutrition of the intervertebral disc. *Spine (Phila Pa 1976)*, 9: 2700-2709.

[23] Nguyen, C., Poiraudeau, S., Rannou, F. (2012). Vertebral subchondral bone. *Osteoporos Int*, S8: 857-860.

[24] Fields, A. J., Sahli, F., Rodriguez, A. G., Lotz, J. C. (2012). Seeing double: a comparison of microstructure, biomechanical function, and adjacent disc health between double- and single-layer vertebral endplates. *Spine (Phila Pa 1976)*, 37: 1310-1317.

[25] Lv, B., Yuan, J., Ding, H., Wan, B., Jiang, Q., Luo, Y., et al. (2019). Relationship between Endplate Defects, Modic Change, Disc Degeneration, and Facet Joint Degeneration in Patients with Low Back Pain. *Biomed Res Int*, 2019: 9369853.

[26] Newell, N., Carpanen, D., Evans, J. H., Pearcy, M. J., Masouros, S. D. (2019). Mechanical Function of the Nucleus Pulposus of the Intervertebral Disc Under High Rates of Loading. *Spine (Phila Pa 1976)*, 44: 1035-1041.

[27] Sun, Z., Luo, Z. J. (2019). Osteoporosis therapies might lead to intervertebral disc degeneration via affecting cartilage endplate. *Med Hypotheses*, 125: 5-7.

[28] Fields, A. J., Ballatori, A., Liebenberg, E. C., Lotz, J. C. (2018). Contribution of the endplates to disc degeneration. *Curr Mol Biol Rep*, 4: 151-160.

[29] Splendiani, A., Bruno, F., Marsecano, C., Arrigoni, F., Di Cesare, E., Barile, A., et al. (2019). Modic I changes size increase from supine to standing MRI correlates with increase in pain intensity in standing position: uncovering the "biomechanical stress" and "active discopathy" theories in low back pain. *Eur Spine J*, 28: 983-992.

[30] Farshad-Amacker, N. A., Hughes, A., Herzog, R. J., Seifert, B., Farshad, M. (2017). The intervertebral disc, the endplates and the vertebral bone marrow as a unit in the process of degeneration. *Eur Radiol*, 27: 2507-2520.

[31] Zhang, J. F., Wang, G. L., Zhou, Z. J., Fang, X. Q., Chen, S., Fan, S. W. (2018). Expression of Matrix Metalloproteinases, Tissue

Inhibitors of Metalloproteinases, and Interleukins in Vertebral Cartilage Endplate. *Orthop Surg*, 10: 306-311.

[32] Määttä, J. H., Rade, M., Freidin, M. B., Airaksinen, O., Karppinen, J., Williams, F. M. K. (2018). Strong association between vertebral endplate defect and Modic change in the general population. *Sci Rep*, 8: 16630.

[33] Zehra, U., Cheung, J. P. Y., Bow, C., Lu, W., Samartzis, D. (2019). Multidimensional vertebral endplate defects are associated with disc degeneration, modic changes, facet joint abnormalities, and pain. *J Orthop Res*, 37: 1080-1089.

[34] Hadjipavlou, A. G., Tzermiadianos, M. N., Bogduk, N., Zindrick, M. R. (2008). The pathophysiology of disc degeneration: a critical review. *J Bone Joint Surg Br*, 90: 1261-1270.

[35] Grignon, B., Grignon, Y., Mainard, D., Braun, M., Netter, P., Roland, J. (2000). The structure of the cartilaginous end-plates in elder people. *Surg Radiol Anat*, 22: 13-19.

[36] Bernick, S., Cailliet, R. (1982). Vertebral end-plate changes with aging of human vertebrae. *Spine*, 7: 97-102.

[37] Pirvu, T., Blanquer, S. B., Benneker, L. M., Grijpma, D. W., Richards, R. G., Alini, M., et al. (2015). A combined biomaterial and cellular approach for annulus fibrosus rupture repair. *Biomaterials*, 42: 11-19.

[38] Sloan, S. R. Jr., Wipplinger, C., Kirnaz, S., Navarro-Ramirez, R., Schmidt, F., McCloskey, D., et al. (2020). Combined nucleus pulposus augmentation and annulus fibrosus repair prevents acute intervertebral disc degeneration after discectomy. *Sci Transl Med*, 12: 2380.

[39] McCulloch, J. A. (1996). Focus issue on lumbar disc herniation: macro- and microdiscectomy. *Spine (Phila Pa 1976)*, 21: 45-56.

[40] Li, X., Dou, Q., Kong, Q. (2016). Repair and Regenerative Therapies of the Annulus Fibrosus of the Intervertebral Disc. *J Coll Physicians Surg Pak*, 26: 138-144.

[41] Vadalà, G., Russo, F., De Strobel, F., Bernardini, M., De Benedictis, G. M., Cattani, C., et al. (2018). Novel stepwise model of

intervertebral disc degeneration with intact annulus fibrosus to test regeneration strategies. *J Orthop Res*, 36: 2460-2468.

[42] Jin, L., Shimmer, A. L., Li, X. (2013). The challenge and advancement of annulus fibrosus tissue engineering. *Eur Spine J*, 22: 1090-1100.

[43] Huang, Y. C., Hu, Y., Li, Z., Luk, K. D. K. (2018). Biomaterials for intervertebral disc regeneration: Current status and looming challenges. *J Tissue Eng Regen Med*, 12: 2188-2202.

[44] Choi, Y., Park, M. H., Lee, K. (2019). Tissue Engineering Strategies for Intervertebral Disc Treatment Using Functional Polymers. *Polymers (Basel)*, 11: 872.

[45] Ashinsky, B. G., Bonnevie, E. D., Mandalapu, S. A., Pickup, S., Wang, C., Han, L., et al. (2020). Intervertebral Disc Degeneration is Associated with Aberrant Endplate Remodeling and Reduced Small Molecule Transport. *J Bone Miner Res*, 4009.

[46] Stich, S., Stolk, M., Girod, P. P., Thomé, C., Sittinger, M., Ringe, J., et al. (2015). Regenerative and immunogenic characteristics of cultured nucleus pulposus cells from human cervical intervertebral discs. *PLoS One*, 10: 0126954.

[47] Naqvi, S. M., Gansau, J., Gibbons, D., Buckley C. T. (2019). In vitro co-culture and ex vivo organ culture assessment of primed and cryopreserved stromal cell microcapsules for intervertebral disc regeneration. *Eur Cell Mater*, 37: 134-152.

[48] Byvaltsev, V. A., Kolesnikov, S. I., Bardonova, L. A., Belykh, E. G., Korytov, L. I., Giers, M. B., et al. (2018). Development of an In Vitro Model of Inflammatory Cytokine Influences on Intervertebral Disk Cells in 3D Cell Culture Using Activated Macrophage-Like THP-1 Cells. *Bull Exp Biol Med*, 166: 151-154.

[49] Chan, S. C., Gantenbein-Ritter, B. (2012). Preparation of intact bovine tail intervertebral discs for organ culture. *J Vis Exp*, 60: 3490.

[50] Haglund, L., Moir, J., Beckman, L., Mulligan, K. R., Jim, B., Ouellet, J. A., et al. (2011). Development of a bioreactor for axially loaded intervertebral disc organ culture. *Tissue Eng Part C Methods*, 17: 1011-1019.

[51] Harris, L., Vangsness, C. T. Jr. (2018). Mesenchymal Stem Cell Levels of Human Spinal Tissues. *Spine (Phila Pa 1976)*, 43: 545-550.

[52] Li, D., Zhu, B., Ding, L., Lu, W., Xu, G., Wu, J. (2014). Role of the mitochondrial pathway in serum deprivation-induced apoptosis of rat endplate cells. *Biochem Biophys Res Commun*, 452: 354-360.

[53] Ariga, K., Yonenobu, K., Nakase, T., Hosono, N., Okuda, S., Meng, W., et al. (2003). Mechanical stress-induced apoptosis of endplate chondrocytes in organ-cultured mouse intervertebral discs: an ex vivo study. *Spine (Phila Pa 1976)*, 28: 1528-1533.

[54] Grant, M. P., Epure, L. M., Bokhari, R., Roughley, P., Antoniou, J., Mwale, F. (2016). Human cartilaginous endplate degeneration is induced by calcium and the extracellular calcium-sensing receptor in the intervertebral disc. *Eur Cell Mater*, 32: 137-151.

[55] Liu, L. T., Huang, B., Li, C. Q., Zhuang, Y., Wang, J., Zhou, Y. (2011). Characteristics of stem cells derived from the degenerated human intervertebral disc cartilage endplate. *PLoS One*, 6: 26285.

[56] Hamilton, D. J., Séguin, C. A., Wang, J., Pilliar, R. M., Kandel, R. A. (2006). Formation of a nucleus pulposus-cartilage endplate construct in vitro. *Biomaterials*, 27: 397-405.

[57] Yin, X., Jiang, L., Yang, J., Cao, L., Dong, J. (2017). Application of biodegradable 3D-printed cage for cervical diseases via anterior cervical discectomy and fusion (ACDF): an in vitro biomechanical study. *Biotechnol Lett*, 39: 1433-1439.

[58] Phelan, K., May, K. M. (2016). Basic Techniques in Mammalian Cell Tissue Culture. *Curr Protoc Toxicol*, 70: 1-22.

[59] Parolin, M., Gawri, R., Mwale, F., Steffen, T., Roughley, P., Antoniou, J., et al. (2010). Development of a whole disc organ culture system to study human intervertebral disc. *Evid Based Spine Care J*, 1: 67-68.

[60] Maroudas, A., Stockwell, R. A., Nachemson, A., Urban, J. (1975). Factors involved in the nutrition of the human lumbar intervertebral disc: cellularity and diffusion of glucose in vitro. *J Anat*, 120: 113-130.

[61] Roughley, P. J. (2004). Biology of intervertebral disc aging and degeneration: involvement of the extracellular matrix. *Spine (Phila Pa 1976)*, 29: 2691-2699.
[62] Antoniou, J., Goudsouzian, N. M., Heathfield, T. F., Winterbottom, N., Steffen, T., Poole, A. R., et al. (1996). The human lumbar endplate. Evidence of changes in biosynthesis and denaturation of the extracellular matrix with growth, maturation, aging, and degeneration. *Spine (Phila Pa 1976)*, 21: 1153-1161.

In: Medical Care
Editor: Brian A. Soileau

ISBN: 978-1-53618-048-0
© 2020 Nova Science Publishers, Inc.

Chapter 5

THE DEGENERATIVE DISEASE OF INTERVERTEBRAL DISC AND SURGICAL RESULTS AFTER MICROSURGICAL DISCECTOMY

Lidija Gradisnik[1,2], *Tomaz Velnar*[2,3,4,*] *and Gorazd Bunc*[4]

[1]Institute of Biomedical Sciences, Medical Faculty Maribor, Maribor, Slovenia
[2]AMEU-ECM Maribor, Maribor, Slovenia
[3]Department of Neurosurgery, University Medical Centre Ljubljana, Ljubljana, Slovenia
[4]Department of Neurosurgery, University Medical Centre Maribor, Ljubljana, Slovenia

ABSTRACT

The degenerative disease of the intervertebral disc and back pain are chronic conditions that are frequently encountered in clinical practice,

---

[*] Corresponding Author's Email: tvelnar@hotmail.com.

especially in young and active population. They are caused by numerous factors and represent an important cause of both morbidity and mortality. Patient comorbidities and numerous associated risk factors may contribute to the onset of the degenerative process. Several factors play a role in the degenerative disc disease, which most commonly affects the nucleus pulposus and eventually influences the biomechanics of the spine. The consequences of the degenerative disc disease are among the main initiative factors for chronic instability of the diseased spinal segments and result in functional disability in both sexes, significantly affecting the quality of living. The mechanisms of the intervertebral disc degeneration and associated factors are presented, as well as our short-term surgical results with microdiscectomy treatment.

Keywords: intervertebral disc, discogenic pain, disc degeneration, surgical treatment, microdiscectomy

INTRODUCTION

The degenerative disease of the intervertebral disc and the back pain are chronic conditions that are caused by numerous factors [1]. They represent an important cause of morbidity and mortality in everyday clinical practice, causing patients to seek both non-operative and operative treatment. The consequences of the degenerative disease of the intervertebral disc are among the main initiative factors for chronic instability of the diseased segments of the spine and for functional disability between both sexes, which significantly affect living quality, especially in young and active population [1, 2]. In the past decades, research has shown that the main etiological factor for the degeneration of the intervertebral disc, in addition to age, gender and long-term exposure to vibrations, is not a strong physical burden associated with particular professions, at least not to the extent it was anticipated. Indeed, physical stresses typical of certain types of occupation and sports activity have a relatively small role in the process of degeneration. On the other hand, these may contribute to the worsening of the already degenerated disc to a great extent. The main reason for the degenerative disc disease are specific interactions between genes and the environment [3, 4]. The influence of heredity is dominant, and the genetic effects on degeneration have been confirmed by the identification of certain genes directly related to the degeneration of the intervertebral plate and acting in conjunction with environmental influences [5, 6].

During the clinical examination, the degenerative disc disease, in the broad sense, may present itself as one of the numerous clinical entities, such as axial back pain, spinal stenosis, myelopathy or radiculopathy, depending on the severity, spinal level and the mechanism of degeneration as well as the affection of the concomitant structures [1, 2]. Patient comorbidities and numerous associated risk factors may contribute to the onset of the degenerative process. The present conservative and surgical treatment techniques may only relieve the pain temporarily in the degenerated spine [1, 2, 7].

The mechanisms of the intervertebral disc degeneration and associated factors are briefly discussed in the text, as well as treatment results with microfenestraion, a microsurgical discectomy according to Caspar technique.

EPIDEMIOLOGICAL CONDITIONS

It is reported that the initial degeneration of intervertebral disc may be present as early as in the adolescence, when 20% of young people have mild signs of the disease. The degeneration of the intervertebral disc tissue starts sooner than that of other muscular and skeletal tissues and is in many cases asymptomatic [8, 9]. With age, however, the incidence rises. In some reports, the degenerative disease of the intervertebral disc may be present in 90% of people; many of them have no signs of the disease [2, 7, 10, 11].

The incidence of low back pain varies among different studies widely. It is the fifth most common cause for the visit to the doctor and affects 7.5% to 37% of patients, based on genetics, gender, age and additional environmental factors. Due to heavier loads and more strenuous motions, disc degeneration usually occurs in the lumbar spine. It affects 10% of male population at the age of 50 years and up to 50% at the age of 70 years. Long lasting pain and movement difficulties are experienced by 10% of patients [1, 2, 7].

Low back pain is strongly connected to the degenerative process of the intervertebral disc [8, 9]. The height of the intervertebral disc gradually falls and the consequence is changed dynamics in the affected segment of the spine. This accelerates the degeneration of other, nearby segments as well as other spinal structures, such as ligaments, joints and muscles. In the long term, this leads to narrowing of the spinal canal with the compression of the neural tissues due to the spinal stenosis, which is the main cause of pain, especially among the elderly. With the increase of elderly population, this problem is gaining significance [9].

THE INTERVERTEBRAL DISC STRUCTURE

The intervertebral disc is an avascular fibrocartilaginous structure, which is located between two neighbouring vertebrae. It is composed of three layers: I) fibrous annulus with its outer and inner part, II) central pulpous nucleus and III) terminal plates [8, 9]. These three parts are all specialized tissues, the latter connecting the disc with the adjacent vertebral bodies. Microscopically, the disc is composed of scarce fibroblast-like cells, located in the extracellular matrix, which accounts for the most of the disc structure. Both cells and matrix are fundamental for normal function of the intervertebral disc [8]. The function of the intervertebral disc is based in providing loading support to the axial skeleton and at the same time allowing the shock absorption and force distribution through the spine during movements, such as extension, flexion, bending and rotation. The fibrous annulus is the most external part of the disc, composed of concentrically arranged fibrocartilaginous lamellae. It is divided into the outer and inner part. The former is mostly composed of type I collagen fibres, oriented radially and in opposite directions throughout concentric lamellae, interposed with interlamellar matrix. The pulpous nucleus is a gelatinous matrix, composed of type II collagen fibres and proteoglycans. Here, scarce nucleus pulposus cells are located, synthesising components of the extracellular matrix and they are responsible for its maintenance. Proteoglycans are most abundant macromolecules in the matrix, containing a core protein with numerous covalently bound glycosaminoglycans and attracting large amounts of water molecules, thus preserving the disc turgor. The loss of proteoglycans is the first act in the disc degeneration cascade, with the consequent loss of water from the nucleus and the change of the disc mechanics [8, 9, 12].

THE PROGRESSION OF DISC DEGENERATION

The border between the annulus of the intervertebral disc and its nucleus becomes more and more pronounced during the growth. Numerous mechanical factors, depending on duration, severity, type and position of load, affect the condition of the intervertebral disc and thus the biological response to these factors [8, 11]. The degenerative processes encompass the structural damage of the intervertebral disc and the changes in the number and composition of cells. With aging and advancing degeneration, the nucleus is primarily affected. It becomes more fibrous and less elastic. Tiny concentric breaks emerge in the outer part of the disc from where they extend into the nucleus. The amount of fibrous tissue rises, the composition and quantity of proteoglycans changes and the number of cells changes due to apoptosis [11, 13-16]. Mechanical, traumatic, genetic and nutritional factors play an important role in the degenerative process. The fibres in the fibrous annulus become increasingly disoriented and the network made of elastin and collagen fibres gradually deteriorates. Cells in the nucleus are affected by apoptosis and later on by necrosis, on the other hand they tend to proliferate excessively. These degenerative cascades are frequent and in an adult intervertebral disc, up to 50% of cells may be necrotic [5, 13, 14].

The main factor in the degeneration of the intervertebral disc is the loss of proteoglycans. These large molecules are degraded to smaller fragments that are lost from disc tissue [13, 17]. The consequence is a fall in the osmotic pressure in the disc matrix and the loss of water molecules, which affects the mechanical properties of the disc. As degenerated intervertebral discs contain less water and have therefore inferior capabilities for sustaining pressure, they bulge and lose height. Proteoglycan loss affects also movement of other molecules into and out of the disc matrix. Serum proteins and cytokines diffuse into the matrix, affecting the cells and accelerating the process of the degeneration [14, 15, 17].

The quantity of the disc collagen and its composition are also connected with the matrix degeneration. The orientation, location and types of collagen fibres are mostly affected, while the effect on the total quantity of collagen is not so pronounced [9, 10]. Old collagen fibres become denatured, although new fibres are being synthesised early in the process of degeneration. The enzyme activity has a significant role in the process of collagen, fibronectin and proteoglycan denaturation and breakdown. Among these, matrix metalloproteinases and cathepsins are essential [10, 14, 18].

The degenerative changes of the intervertebral disc are connected to the damage of nearby structures, such as ligaments, joints and vertebral muscles. This leads to functional changes and greater susceptibility to injuries [9, 18]. Due to load, a degenerated intervertebral disc is lower than normal and apophyseal joints need to bear higher loads. The consequence is osteoarthritic degeneration. The strength of yellow ligaments decreases, which leads to their hypertrophy and protrusion of the ligaments into the spinal canal with consequent narrowing and compression of neural structures. The causes of pain in the course of the degenerative process are complex and in many cases a fair combination of structural and mechanical deformation as well as activity of inflammatory mediators [19]. Frequently, spinal nerve radices are involved in the degenerative cascade, which causes chronic pain mainly due to their compression and partly due to the ingrowths of tiny neural endings into the degenerated disc and their activation due to the constant release of inflammatory mediators [9, 19].

Herniated and prolapsed discs are among the most frequent reasons for presentation to the orthopaedist or neurosurgeon. A herniation is bulging of the disc due to partial or complete rupture of the outer fibrous annulus. The bulging may involve anterior, posterolateral or posterior direction. The last two directions are particularly important as they cause compression of the neural structures in the vertebral canal [20]. Occasionally, spontaneous resorption of the disc may occur, leading to improvement or even cessation of lumbar pain [21]. Although disc herniation is most commonly caused due to mechanical injury and consequent rupture of the fibrous annulus, some extent of initial degeneration is necessary in order to allow the pulpous nucleus to herniate through fibrous bands of annulus into the vertebral canal. For a healthy disc to rupture, an enormous force is necessary. In many cases, the terminal plates of vertebrae fail sooner than the fibrous belt [4, 6, 13, 22, 23].

FACTORS INFLUENCING THE DEGENERATIVE PROCESS

Degeneration due to Nutritional Disorders of the Disc

One of the important reasons for the degenerative process is also nutritional disorder of the intervertebral disc [24]. For normal function and structure of the disc, the cells need sufficient nutritional supply. A disc is avascular structure and its supply depends mainly on diffusion. Capillaries arising in the vertebral bodies extend only to the subchondral area of the disc terminal plate. This means that gasses and nutrients must diffuse through extracellular matrix in order to reach the cells. A fall in nutritional supply causes a fall in oxygen quantity and a rise in lactate concentration with consequent pH alteration, affecting the cell function and synthesis of extracellular matrix. In the long term, this leads to degenerative process [23-26].

Mechanical Stress

Abnormal mechanical loads and microscopical injuries lead to disc degeneration through faster wear and tear of both acellular and cellular components, involving the processes described earlier. The common consequence is chronic pain [27]. The most important risk factors involve heavy physical labour, obesity, smoking (through the atherosclerosis of minute vessels that supply the terminal plates), lack of physical activity and inappropriate flexed posture [17, 27, 28].

Genetic Factors

There is also a genetic basis for the degenerative process of the intervertebral disc. Certain genetic polymorphisms for matrix molecules define the integrity of the extracellular matrix and these polymorphisms may also influence the course of the degenerative process [26, 29]. Mutations in genes coding for matrix molecules lead to alterations of matrix morphology, consequently affecting the function and biochemical processes of the disc. However, genes alone are not the only reasons for disc disease as environmental factors are also involved, showing that intervertebral disc degeneration is probably a multifactorial disease [30-32].

Bacterial Infection of the Intervertebral Disc

The exact pathobiology of degenerative disc disease is still unknown [31, 32]. As discussed, numerous factors play a role in the degeneration, such as genetics, vascular aspects, mechanical stress, inflammatory and biochemical changes. One of recently described agents that may start the degenerative process are also bacteria. It has been proposed, according to some studies, that intervertebral disc degeneration might be initiated by a long-lasting low-grade infection, eventually leading to the disc prolapse and herniation [33]. The *Propionibacterium acnes* is the most commonly isolated infectious agent, which may be the principal cause for the disc disease. Some studies concerning the bacteriology of the intervertebral discs have been conducted and the results were contradictory [33, 34]. Although the positive disc cultures may have resulted from specimen contamination after disc removal, on the other hand, the degeneration processes were stopped or slowed by antibiotic treatment. It is still not known whether the genesis of disc degeneration originates in the immune system and repeated episodes of injury and reparation that could eventually culminate to the progressive tissue damage [33-36].

MICRODISCECTOMY RESULTS AT OUR CLINIC

Our neurosurgical department is heavily involved in the treatment of spinal degenerative diseases. Among versatile pathology, disc herniation are one of the most frequently encountered. The back pain and especially radicular pain resulting from nerve compression represent an important cause of morbidity, especially in the active population, regardless of the age.

When caused by a herniated disc of various degrees, the treatment of lumbar radicular compressive syndromes usually encompasses discectomy and/or foraminotomy, thus relieving the compressed nerve root. Microsurgical discectomy and the success of microsurgical procedure according to the Caspar technique are presented below.

Patients and Methods

In the prospective study in 2016, 146 patients were included. All of them suffered from the lumbar radiculopathy due to a herniated disc induced nerve compression. The diagnostic imaging involved dynamic x-rays, computed tomography (CT) and magnetic resonance imaging (MRI) in order to diagnose and to conform the clinical predictions. The X-rays was done only in those patents, where lumbar instability was expected. When confirmed, these patients were excluded from the study, as were those with lumbar spinal canal stenosis and pure foraminal stenosis.

In the included population, conservative treatment was not successful and operation was recommended. A standard Caspar microdiscectomy (microfenestration) was performed, that has been used is in everyday clinical practice at our clinical department [37]. Briefly, the patient was positioned prone or in the genupectoral position with the care taken not to compress the abdomen and consequently cause the epidural venous congestion, which may lead to the increased haemorrhage during the procedure.

Preoperatively, fluoroscopy was used to determine the level of the discectomy, by inserting a spinal needle vertically to the inferior edge of the affected disc. A skin incision of about 3cm in length was done at the lateral margin of the labelled spinous processes, the lumbar fascia was exposed and cut in a linear manner about 1cm to 1.5cm from the midline. The paraspinal muscles were subperiostally detached and retracted laterally. The Caspar retractor was then inserted and positioned properly, so that the interlaminar space was seen. Under the operating microscope, a limited resection of the lower quarter of the upper lamina and medial portion of the medial facet joint was performed. The yellow ligament was visualised and removed and the dural sac with the nerve root in question was identified underneath. After the nerve root was detached from the herniation and gently medialised, the herniated disc was exposed. The overlaying longitudinal ligament was incised and the disc space was evacuated using curetes and rongeurs. The disc space and wound was washed and the closure the fascia, subcutaneous tissue and skin followed [37, 38].

The follow up of our patients was evaluated from 1 to 3 years after the operation, the average evaluation time was 15 months. Of 146 patients, 49.5% were men and 51.5% were women. The average age of the studied population was 49.05 years (range 19 to 74 years) with the average age in men 46.3 years and in women 51.8 years. The patients were followed up regularly after the operation, initially after 3 to 4 months and then after one year at earliest and after 3 years at latest.

The success of the operative treatment was evaluated with the Maribor scale (MB-scale) and with the Oswestry disability index, where the dailiy activities, satisfaction with the operative treatment and the postoperative pan were evaluated [39].

Results

The diagnosis of radiculopathy due to a herniated disc of various severity was confirmed in all of our patients. In some, the foraminal stenosis was a concomitant pathology, addressing also this entity during the operation. The percentage of patients with their respective pathology and the levels of pathology are shown in Tables 1 and 2.

Short-term results of surgery were evaluated during the first follow up, 3 to 4 months after the operation. The postoperative pain was significantly reduced in 89.8% patients. The pain was persisting unchanged in 7.9% patents and was evaluated as worse in 2.3% patients. Overall, the operation was successful in 97.7% patients.

Table 1. The percentage of treated patients and their respective lumbar pathology

Pathology	Percentage of patients
Herniated disc	32.1
Ruptured hernia	25.3
Ruptured hernia with free fragment	39.7
Herniated disc with foraminal stenosis	2.9

Table 2. The incidence of various lumbar disc herniations

Level of pathology	Percentage of patients
L5-S1	56.7
L4-L5	34.3
L3-L4	6.4
L2-L3	2.6

The rest of them reported a worsening of the radicular pain and this group was evaluated by MRI. Those diagnosed with a recidive of lumbar hernia were operated on again. The quality of life has improved in 87.5% patients and was unchanged or worse in 12.5% patients. No difference in treatment outcome between male and female patents has been observed.

Long-term results were evaluated 1 to 3 years postoperatively. These revealed an excellent treatment outcome in 68%, good outcome in 27%, fair in 2% and poor in 3% of patients. One patient died one month after the operation due to unrelated reasons and was not included in the final assessment. Thus, the total result was satisfactory in 94%. There was no difference in treatment outcome between male and female patents. A poor outcome included recidives of the herniated disc at the same level (in 2.4% of the operated patients) and local complications, such as fibrosis of the nerve root, infection (spondylodiscitis) and complications in wound healing.

Discussion

The degenerative disease of the intervertebral disc and back pain are chronic conditions representing an important cause of morbidity, especially in the active population [27, 28]. The treatment of lumbar radicular compressive syndromes usually encompasses discectomy and/or foraminotomy, thus relieving the compressed nerve root. Microsurgical discectomy and the success of microsurgical procedure according to the Caspar technique is a well-established mode of treatment in the neurosurgical and orthopaedic clinical practice [37, 38]. The operation is relatively simple and quick and bears a successful treatment outcome in comparison to other, older techniques and approaches. However, it is not without risks and suitable only for a rather limited surgical approach in the treatment for intervertebral disc herniation or faraminotomy. Exactly the same indications were also used in our group of patients. The short- and long term results of microsurgical approach showed the efficiency especially in the early postoperative period, which was attributed, on our opinion, particularly to the limited surgical approach. The skin wound, muscle detachment and bone (laminar) removal was minimal and the postoperative pain and wound healing accordingly, which enabled a fast recovery of patients, earlier mobilisation, lower analgesic intake and quicker return to normal daily activities. On the other hand, the pain, healing course and complications are more often encountered with wider surgical approaches for treatment of intervertebral disc herniations. The results of our microdiscectomy series can be compared with similar results elsewhere according to the international criteria (88% to 98% treatment sucess). The successfulness of the microsurgical method is due to gentle tissue handling, especially with respect to the nerve structures in the spinal canal and considerably smaller injury of muscles and bone [40-42]. This is achieved by better visibility and field magnification with the operative microscope. The good results of microdiscectomy affirm this technique as a useful method in clinical practice.

CONCLUSION

The degenerative disease of the intervertebral disc remains a significant health problem, still not understood and solved sufficiently [43, 44]. Besides standard conservative and surgical treatment, techniques of regenerative therapy are very promising, although most of them still in the experimental phase [41-44]. Regenerative therapy aims to restore the degenerated disc matrix by two approaches: with growth factors enhancing extracellular matrix synthesis by the disc cells and with agents inhibiting cytokines that normally cause the loss of matrix [41-43].

REFERENCES

[1] Maniadakis, N., Gray, A. (2000). The economic burden of back pain in the UK. *Pain,* 84: 95 - 103.

[2] Cheung, K. M., Karppinen, J., Chan, D., Ho, D. W., Song, Y. Q., Sham, P. et al. (2009). Prevalence and pattern of lumbar magnetic resonance imaging changes in a population study of one thousand forty-three individuals. *Spine,* 34: 934 - 940.

[3] Miller, J., Schmatz, C., Schultz, A. (1998). Lumbar disc degeneration: Correlation with age, sex, and spine level in 600 autopsy specimens. *Spine,* 13:173 - 178.

[4] Setton, L. A., Chen, J. (2006). Mechanobiology of the intervertebral disc and relevance to disc degeneration. *J. Bone Joint Surg. Am.,* 88: 52 - 57.

[5] Fearing, B. V., Hernandez, P. A., Setton, L. A., Chahine, N. O. (2018). Mechanotransduction and cell biomechanics of the intervertebral disc. *JOR Spine,* 1:1026.

[6] Manchikanti, L., Derby, R., Benyamin, R. M., Helm, S., Hirsch, J. A. (2009). A systematic review of mechanical lumbar disc decompression with nucleoplasty. *Pain Physician,* 12: 561 - 572.

[7] Kanayama, M., Togawa, D., Takahashi, C., Terai, T., Hashimoto, T. (2009). Cross-sectional magnetic resonance imaging study of lumbar disc degeneration in 200 healthy individuals. *J. Neurosurg. Spine,* 4:501 - 507.

[8] Cheung, K. M., Orlansky, A. S., Sen, K., Elliot, D. M. (2009). Reduced nucleus pulposus glycosaminoglycan content alters intervertebral disc dynamic viscoelastic mechanics. *J. Biomech.,* 42: 1941 - 1946.

[9] Colombini, A., Lombardi, G., Corsi, M. M., Banfi, G. (2008). Pathophysiology of the human intervertebral disc. *Int. J. Biochem. Cell Biol.,* 40: 837 - 842.

[10] Kalichman, L., Kim, D. H., Li, L., Guermazi, A., Hunter, D. J. (2010). Computed tomography-evaluated features of spinal degeneration: prevalence, intercorrelation, and association with self-reported low back pain. *Spine J.,* 10: 200 - 208.

[11] Łebkowski, W. J. (2002). Autopsy evaluation of the extent of degeneration of the lumbar intervertebral discs. *Pol. Merkur Lekarski,* 13: 188 - 190.

[12] Cannata, F., Vadalà, G., Ambrosio, L., Fallucca, S., Napoli, N., Papalia, R. et al. (2020). Intervertebral disc degeneration: A focus on obesity and type 2 diabetes. *Diabetes Metab. Res. Rev.,* 36:3224.

[13] Roughley, P. J. (2004). Biology of intervertebral disc aging and degeneration: involvement of the extracellular matrix. *Spine,* 29: 2691 - 2699.

[14] Inoue, N., Espinoza Orías, A. A. (2011). Biomechanics of intervertebral disk degeneration. *Orthop. Clin. North Am.,* 42: 487 - 499.

[15] Jarman, J. P., Arpinar, V. E., Baruah, D., Klein, A. P., Maiman, D. J., Muftuler, L. T. (2015). Intervertebral disc height loss demonstrates the threshold of major pathological changes during degeneration. *Eur. Spine J.,* 24: 1944 - 1950.

[16] Hsieh, A. H., Twomey, J. D. (2010). Cellular mechanobiology of the intervertebral disc: New directions and approaches. *J. Biomech.,* 43: 137 - 145.

[17] Singh, K., Masuda, K., Thonar, E. J., An, H. S., Cs-Szabo, G. (2009). Age-related changes in the extracellular matrix of nucleus pulposus and anulus fibrosus of human intervertebral disc. *Spine,* 34: 10 - 16.

[18] Grignon, B., Grignon, Y., Mainard, D., Braun, M., Netter, P., Roland, J. (2000). The structure of the cartilaginous end-plates in elder people. *Surg. Radiol. Anat.,* 22: 13 - 19.

[19] Bernick, S., Cailliet, R. (1982). Vertebral end-plate changes with aging of human vertebrae. *Spine,* 7: 97 - 102.

[20] Veres, S. P., Robertson, P. A., Broom, N. D. (2009). The morphology of acute disc herniation: a clinically relevant model defining the role of flexion. *Spine,* 34: 2288 - 2296.

[21] Chang, C. W., Lai, P. H., Yip, C. M., Hsu, S. S. (2009). Spontaneous regression of lumbar herniated disc. *J. Chin. Med. Assoc.,* 72: 650 - 653.

[22] Millisdotter, M., Strömqvist, B., Jönsson, B. (2003). Proximal neuromuscular impairment in lumbar disc herniation: a prospective controlled study. *Spine,* 28: 1281 - 1289.

[23] Hadjipavlou, A. G., Tzermiadianos, M. N., Bogduk, N., Zindrick, M. R. (2008). The pathophysiology of disc degeneration: a critical review. *J. Bone Joint Surg. Br.,* 90: 1261 - 1270.
[24] Urban, J. P., Smith, S., Fairbank, J. C. (2004). Nutrition of the intervertebral disc. *Spine,* 29: 2700 - 2709.
[25] Grunhagen, T., Wilde, G., Soukane, D. M., Shirazi-Adl, S. A., Urban, J. P. (2006). Nutrient supply and intervertebral disc metabolism. *J. Bone Joint Surg. Am.,* 88: 30 - 35.
[26] Zhang, Y., Sun, Z., Liu, J., Guo, X. (2008). Advances in susceptibility genetics of intervertebral degenerative disc disease. *Int. J. Biol. Sci.,* 4: 283 - 290.
[27] Battié, M. C., Videman, T., Parent, E. (2004). Lumbar disc degeneration: epidemiology and genetic influences. *Spine,* 29: 2679 - 2690.
[28] Luoma, K., Riihimäki, H., Raininko, R., Luukkonen, R., Lamminen, A., Viikari-Juntura, E. (1998). Lumbar disc degeneration in relation to occupation. *Scand. J. Work Environ. Health,* 24: 358 - 366.
[29] Matsui, H., Kanamori, M., Ishihara, H., Yudoh, K., Naruse, Y., Tsuji, H. (1998). Familial predisposition for lumbar degenerative disc disease. A case-control study. *Spine,* 23: 1029 - 1034.
[30] Battié, M. C., Videman, T., Levälahti, E., Gill, K., Kaprio, J. (2008). Genetic and environmental effects on disc degeneration by phenotype and spinal level: a multivariate twin study. *Spine,* 33: 2801 - 2808.
[31] Hubert, M. G., Vadala, G., Sowa, G., Studer, R. K., Kang, J. D. (2008). Gene therapy for the treatment of degenerative disk disease. *J. Am. Acad. Orthop. Surg.,* 16: 312 - 319.
[32] Chan, D., Song, Y., Sham, P., Cheung, K. M. (2006). Genetics of disc degeneration. *Eur. Spine J.,* 15: S317 - 325.
[33] Arndt, J., Charles, Y. P., Koebel, C., Bogorin, I., Steib, J. P. (2012). Bacteriology of degenerated lumbar intervertebral disks. *J. Spinal Disord. Tech.,* 25: 211 - 216.
[34] Delogu, G., Zumbo, A., Fadda, G. (2012). Microbiological and immunological diagnosis of tuberculous spondylodiscitis. *Eur. Rev. Med. Pharmacol. Sci.,* 16: 73 - 78.

[35] Gasbarrini, A., Boriani, L., Salvadori, C., Mobarec, S., Kreshak, J., Nanni, C. et al. (2012). Biopsy for suspected spondylodiscitis. *Eur. Rev. Med. Pharmacol. Sci.,* 16: 26 - 34.

[36] Agarwal, V., Golish, S. R., Alamin, T. F. (2011). Bacteriologic culture of excised intervertebral disc from immunocompetent patients undergoing single level primary lumbar microdiscectomy. *J. Spinal Disord. Tech.,* 24: 397 - 400.

[37] Papavero, L., Caspar, W. (1993). The lumbar microdiscectomy. *Acta Orthop. Scand. Suppl.,* 251: 34 - 37.

[38] Caspar, W. (1985). The microsurgical technique for herniated lumbar disc operation. *Aesculap Scientific Information,* WI-20, Ed 111.

[39] Bunc, G., Strnad, S. (1998). Dolgoročni rezultati mikrodiscektomij v primerjavi s kratkoročnimi. *Zdrav. Vestn.,* 67: 519 - 524.

[40] Ruan, D., He, Q., Ding, Y., Hou, L., Li, J., Luk, K. D. (2007). Intervertebral disc transplantation in the treatment of degenerative spine disease: a preliminary study. *Lancet,* 369: 993 - 999.

[41] Bron, J. L., Helder, M. N., Meisel, H. J., Van Royen, B. J., Smit, T. H. (2009). Repair, regenerative and supportive therapies of the annulus fibrosus: achievements and challenges. *Eur. Spine J.,* 18: 301 - 313.

[42] Alini, M., Roughley, P. J., Antoniou, J., Stoll, T., Aebi, M. (2002). A biological approach to treating disc degeneration: not for today, but maybe for tomorrow. *Eur. Spine J.,* 11: 215 - 220.

[43] Endres, M., Abbushi, A., Thomale, U. W., Cabraja, M., Kroppenstedt, S. N., Morawietz, L. et al. (2010). Intervertebral disc regeneration after implantation of a cell-free bioresorbable implant in a rabbit disc degeneration model. *Biomaterials,* 31: 5836 - 5841.

[44] Nakashima, S., Matsuyama, Y., Takahashi, K., Satoh, T., Koie, H., Kanayama, K. et al. (2009). Regeneration of intervertebral disc by the intradiscal application of cross-linked hyaluronate hydrogel and cross-linked chondroitin sulfate hydrogel in a rabbit model of intervertebral disc injury. *Biomed. Mater. Eng.,* 19: 421 - 429.

INDEX

A

adverse effects, 22
aerobic exercise, 7
age, 9, 11, 36, 39, 42, 44, 46, 48, 53, 61, 64, 66, 73, 74, 96, 97, 103, 104, 108
anxiety, 5, 19
anxiety disorder, 19
apoptosis, 78, 93, 99
apraxia, 24, 36, 52, 53
arthroplasty, 78
articular cartilage, 74
atherosclerosis, 102
autism, ix, 24, 29, 42, 49, 51, 53, 63, 70
autonomic nervous system, 53
axial skeleton, 98

B

back pain, xi, 24, 73, 76, 88, 90, 95, 96, 97, 98, 103, 106, 107, 108
biomechanics, xi, 88, 89, 96, 108
body weight, 45, 46
bone, 46, 50, 63, 74, 75, 76, 77, 90, 107
bone marrow, 75, 76, 90

C

cartilage, 74, 75, 77, 84, 87, 90, 93
cartilaginous, x, xi, 72, 74, 75, 76, 79, 81, 82, 83, 84, 85, 86, 87, 91, 93, 109
cell culture, xi, 72, 78, 80, 81, 82, 85, 86, 87
cell death, 73
cell isolation, xi, 72, 85, 86
cell lines, 86
central modulation, 2, 5
central nervous system, vii, ix, 2, 4, 5, 22, 23
cerebral palsy, 42, 48, 66, 69, 70
children, 10, 24, 29, 36, 42, 45, 46, 50, 53, 54, 62, 64, 66, 68, 69, 70
chondrocyte, xi, 72, 73, 79, 85, 87
chondrocytes, vi, vii, x, xi, 71, 72, 78, 79, 81, 82, 84, 85, 86, 87, 93
chondroitin sulfate, 111
chronic fatigue, viii, 1, 3, 22
cognitive function, 20, 36, 56
collagen, x, 72, 74, 75, 77, 81, 83, 84, 87, 98, 99, 100

cytokines, 77, 100, 107
cytoplasm, 83, 86
cytoskeleton, 81

D

degenerative conditions, 89
degenerative disc disease, vi, x, xi, 71, 72, 73, 76, 77, 78, 79, 96, 97, 102, 110
diagnostic criteria, viii, 2, 3, 9, 48
disability, xi, 54, 73, 96, 104
disc degeneration, xi, 72, 73, 75, 76, 77, 78, 84, 90, 91, 96, 97, 99, 101, 102, 103, 108, 109, 110, 111
discogenic pain, 96
discomfort, 7, 42, 55
discs, 88, 89, 92, 93, 100, 102, 108
disk disease, 110
dopamine, 26, 27
dopamine agonist, 26
dopaminergic, 22

E

endplate, vi, vii, x, xi, 71, 72, 73, 74, 75, 76, 77, 78, 79, 81, 82, 83, 84, 85, 86, 87, 88, 90, 91, 92, 93, 94
exercise, 58, 64, 66
exercise programs, 58
extracellular matrix, 76, 77, 84, 94, 98, 101, 102, 107, 109

F

fibromyalgia, v, vii, viii, 1, 2, 3, 8, 9, 12, 13, 14, 15, 17, 18, 20, 21, 22, 23, 24, 25, 26, 27, 28, 29, 30, 31
fibrosis, 89, 106
fibrositis, 3, 29, 30, 31
fibrous tissue, 99

flexibility, 60, 74
flexor, 46, 62

G

GMFM score, v, ix, 33, 34
gross motor function, vii, ix, x, 34, 35, 36, 37, 42, 43, 47, 48, 52, 53, 54, 55, 56, 57, 58, 59, 61, 62, 63, 64, 65, 68, 69

H

herniated, 103, 104, 105, 106, 109, 111
hypersensitivity, viii, 2, 6, 8, 14, 18, 21, 52, 63
hyperventilation, 35

I

impairments, vii, ix, 34, 51, 54, 67
improvements, 58, 62, 63, 64, 65
in vitro, vii, x, xi, 72, 73, 78, 79, 84, 87, 93
in vivo, 85, 87
inflammatory mediators, 77, 100
interdisciplinary treatment, 52
intervention, 38, 41, 47, 48, 53, 54, 55, 56, 58, 60, 61, 63, 64, 65
intervertebral disc, vii, x, xi, 72, 73, 74, 75, 76, 77, 78, 79, 84, 85, 87, 88, 89, 90, 91, 92, 93, 94, 95, 96, 97, 98, 99, 100, 101, 102, 106, 107, 108, 109, 110, 111

J

joints, 21, 98, 100

K

knees, 43
kyphosis, 35, 44

L

laminar, 107
locomotor, ix, 34
lumbar radiculopathy, 103

M

magnetic resonance imaging (MRI), 4, 26, 30, 73, 88, 90, 103, 106, 108
matrix, 73, 76, 77, 84, 87, 98, 99, 100, 101, 102, 107
matrix metalloproteinase, 77, 100
mental health, viii, 2, 11, 16, 18
mental illness, 19
mesenchymal stem cells, 78
metabolism, 63, 84, 110
microcephaly, 34, 52
microdiscectomy, vii, xi, 91, 96, 103, 107, 111
microsurgical discectomy, vi, 95, 97
modified GMFM score, 34
mood disorder, 3
mood swings, viii, 2
morbidity, xi, 96, 103, 106
morphology, 76, 77, 81, 83, 86, 102, 109
mortality, xi, 96
motivation, 50, 64, 67
motor control, 42, 56, 70
motor skills, 37, 42, 65
muscle relaxant, 7
muscle strength, 60
muscles, 3, 21, 98, 100, 104, 107
musculoskeletal, viii, 1, 3, 55
musculoskeletal system, 55

N

nerve, 45, 46, 75, 100, 103, 104, 106
nervous system, 5, 22, 23
neurological disorder(s), v, ix, 33, 34, 35, 52, 65
neurological rehabilitation, 52, 53, 54, 67
neurotransmitters, 4, 22
nitrogen, 82
non-steroidal anti-inflammatory drugs, 7
normal development, 46, 54
nutrient(s), x, 72, 75, 78, 101
nutrition, 75, 84, 93

O

obesity, 73, 102, 109
occupational therapy, 69
osmotic pressure, 76, 99
osteoporosis, 46

P

pain, viii, x, 1, 3, 7, 10, 19, 21, 22, 23, 25, 26, 27, 29, 31, 35, 52, 73, 75, 90, 91, 96, 97, 98, 100, 101, 102, 103, 105, 106, 107
pain perception, 4, 21, 23
paralysis, x, 52
pathology, 79, 85, 88, 103, 105
pathophysiological, vii, viii, 2, 3, 21, 22, 78
pathophysiology, 91, 110
peripheral nervous system, viii, 2, 3, 21, 34
physical activity, 63, 102
physical characteristics, 55
physical fitness, 50, 70
physical health, viii, 2, 11, 16, 18, 20
physical mechanisms, 73
physical therapy, 7, 58
physiology, vii, ix, 2, 22, 85

Q

quality of life, viii, 2, 5, 8, 10, 16, 17, 18, 19, 20, 23, 27, 28, 29, 35, 106

R

radiculopathy, 97, 105
regression, 36, 42, 44, 52, 55, 63, 64, 109
rehabilitation, 54, 61, 65
repair, 78, 84, 88, 89, 91
reparation, 92, 103
Rett syndrome, v, vii, ix, 34, 38, 47, 48, 49, 50, 51, 52, 53, 65, 66, 67, 68, 70
rheumatic diseases, 20
rheumatoid arthritis, 28
risk factors, xi, 73, 96, 97, 102

S

scoliosis, 35, 36, 44, 46, 49, 66
sensitivity, viii, 2, 4, 6, 12, 13, 14, 15, 18, 21, 22, 25, 26
sensitization, 10, 14, 18, 29
sensory hypersensitivity, 2, 6, 8, 18, 25
sensory integration, v, 1, 2, 5, 8, 9, 23, 27, 28, 29, 31, 69
sensory modalities, 20
sensory system(s), 4, 5, 12, 20, 56
speech, vii, ix, 34, 42, 51, 53, 54, 63
spinal cord, ix, 52
spinal fusion, 78
spinal stenosis, 97, 98
spine, xi, 44, 62, 73, 85, 96, 97, 98, 108, 111
Statistical Package for the Social Sciences (SPSS software), 38, 58
stenosis, 103, 105
stimulus, 6, 12, 13, 14, 15, 18
stress, viii, 2, 4, 19, 22, 73, 75, 90, 93
surgical treatment, 96, 97, 107
sympathetic nervous system, 75
symptoms, viii, ix, 1, 3, 7, 9, 18, 19, 22, 23, 44, 51

T

techniques, 42, 43, 54, 61, 78, 97, 106, 107
therapeutic approaches, 85
therapeutic effects, 69
therapy, 7, 30, 37, 39, 40, 48, 62, 63, 65, 68, 69, 70, 78, 107, 110
tissue, x, 21, 72, 76, 77, 78, 79, 80, 85, 86, 92, 97, 99, 103, 107
tissue engineering, 92
treatment, vii, ix, xi, 7, 10, 19, 23, 24, 25, 27, 34, 35, 41, 42, 50, 52, 55, 57, 58, 61, 67, 68, 69, 72, 78, 84, 87, 96, 97, 103, 104, 106, 107, 110, 111

V

vertebrae, 74, 84, 91, 98, 101, 109
vestibular system, 14, 21
visual stimuli, 18
visual system, 14, 21

W

walking, 42, 45, 46, 48, 50, 58, 63, 66, 68
wound healing, 106, 107

X

x-rays, 103